D0816212

PREGNANT MAN

PREGNANT MAN

HOW NATURE MAKES
FATHERS
OUT OF MEN

GORDON CHURCHWELL

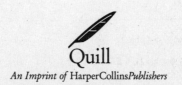

Quill
An Imprint of HarperCollinsPublishers

For my parents, who gave me life,
and Julie and Olivia, who help me live it

First Quill edition published 2001.

Designed by Elliott Beard

The Library of Congress has catalogued the hardcover edition as follows:

Churchwell, Gordon.
    Expecting: one man's uncensored memoir of pregnancy/ Gordon Churchwell.—1st ed.
        p. cm.
    ISBN 0-06-039345-9
        1. Pregnancy—Popular works. 2. Pregnancy—Humor. 3. Pregnant women—Relations with men. I. Title.

RG525.c48 2000
618.2'4—dc21   99-089720

ISBN 0-06-098839-8 (pbk.)

01 02 03 04 05 ❖/RRD 10 9 8 7 6 5 4 3 2 1

CONTENTS

CONTENTS

ACKNOWLEDGMENTS

I am grateful to many people for the opportunity to write this, my first book. Foremost are my agent, Elaine Markson, and my editor, Laura Yorke. Elaine nurtured and supported me from the moment my proposal landed on her desk. Her telephone calls are better than breathing oxygen. Laura's enthusiasm, commitment, and vision sustained me for two and a half years, and her brilliant editing brought out the very best in me. I would also like to thank the following wonderful people at Harper-Collins for making me feel at home and contributing their care, professionalism and many talents to the publishing process: Gail Winston, Bridget Sweeney, Sue Llewellyn, Maggie McMahon, Chris McKerrow, and Craig Herman.

Everyone needs to get started, and so special thanks go out to Andy and Alex Postman, who helped me take the first steps on the long road by being so generous with their time and sparkling intelligence, and that first important phone call.

The business of caring for mothers and delivering babies is a passionate one, and as well as thanking the following people for contributing their knowledge and expertise to this book, I also want to say how much I admire them for their dedication and professionalism: Barbara Scofield, Jan Wenk, Erica Lyons, Julie Tupler, Linda Ware, and Adam Romoff.

Since science is so critical to the book being what it is, I would like to thank the following scientists for generously sharing their work and ideas: Anne Storey, Robert Elwood, Mack Lipkin, Donald Symons, Laura Rival, Ed Hagen, and Wenda Trevathan.

Because someone had to help me understand the science, much gratitude goes out to the following scientists who took the time to share their knowledge and contacts, as well as educating me with great congeniality of spirit: Tom Insel, David Gubernick, C. Sue Carter, Gareth Leng, Alison Fleming, Craig Kinsley, Jay Rosenblatt, Cort Pedersen, Terrence Deacon, Connie Sutton, Alma Gottlieb, Philip Romero, Colin Ingram, and John Russell.

From the world of experience I would like to thank the following people for bravely sharing their stories and thoughts with me: Jamie Silverstein, John Emy, Giovanna Gould, Tom Hirschi, Jane Smillie, Alon Gratsch, Rick Balmaseda, Guy Gleysteen, Mary Hogue, Tony Dunaif, Walter Garschagen, Matthew Deserio, Tim Button, Bob Bozic, David Shenk, Howard Lew, Ippolita Rostagno, and Leigh Giurlando. Also, special thanks to Robin Preisler and Allen Sundstrom, without whose encouragement we would never have had a child in the first place.

The following readers provided me with great encouragement and course corrections along the way: Noelle Oxenhandler, Beth Cody Kimmel, Liz Gilbert, Gwen Dunaif, Melissa Ptacek, and Jill Herzig.

Finally it's important to go back some years and thank a few people who made a real difference in my life by making sure I learned how to think and write: Don Berry, Hank Payne, Margaret Maurer, Gabe Winter, and Edith Kern.

MONTH ONE

IN THE BEGINNING . . .

Ambivalence doesn't even begin to do justice to what is happening to me.

It's 6:30 A.M. My wife is peeing on what looks like a scale model of the spaceship from *2001: A Space Odyssey.* It's an early pregnancy test called something like First Alert, or Early Response, some name that sounds like a smoke detector or a piece of EMS equipment. I should remember the name, because I went to a lot of trouble to be the one to go out and buy it, so that I could show how positive I was about our plans to have a baby, to telegraph, to signal what a sensitive and "proactive" partner I was going to be.

I know as we peer at the little window that I am going to be required to display some emotion, whether the window remains light mauve, indicating negative, or turns darker mauve, indicating positive.

We synch up for a moment to decide with nervous giggles that whoever designed this test is either a sadist or a moron. Why can't the little window say "Yes" or "No," "Win" or "Lose," "Continue with Your Perfect Life" or "Risk Everything"?

With both of us raptly looking on, the window darkens. Mauve, dark mauve is storming across the window like a Panzer division. It's definite. Mauve has asserted itself. The dye is cast.

My wife looks up from our little science project, a smile radiating upward and outward from her lips, carried on a hundred million capillaries of happiness. "Well, what do you think? Aren't you happy?" she asks me.

I'm thinking: "Isn't that what Marie Curie said to her husband when she discovered radioactivity?"

Let's just say my reaction is a little more subtle, a little more complex. What I'm really worried about is the fact that I can't seem to summon up any emotion at all. I know I'm supposed to feel something, but inside my emotional self is on a ventilator. To top it all off, I'm having an out-of-body experience like you read about as you're checking out of the supermarket. You know, those near-death testimonials: "There I was hovering over the O.R. while they operated desperately, trying to save my life." I'm thinking, perhaps the shock of all this has actually killed me.

I'm about to turn toward the "long tunnel of light" when I notice that what I've been watching is my expression reflected in the bathroom mirror. One look at my blank face and I realize that I have to do something to save myself. I pull an Ali "rope-a-dope" and pull Julie toward me with a hug, mumbling with as much conviction as I can muster, "Yes doll, of course I'm happy. This is *so* wonderful."

I glance at ourselves clinching in the mirror. Julie, her head tucked into my shoulder, is the very picture of mother-to-be bliss. And me? The expectant zombie-father. I give myself the eye. Whatever part of me is still alive knows I'm in deep trouble.

•   •   •

"Women are creatures of biology and destiny with philosophies synchronized to a progressive vision of history with the same certainty as their uteruses are timed to the cycles of nature and the clock of the cosmos.

"Men are ahistorical, transitory, emotion-deferring, future-obsessed creatures whose only bonds with biology are hunger and libido—mobile GI tracts with egos and penises.

"What makes women women makes them relationship-driven, life-perpetuating, and family-centered.

"What makes men men makes them self-intoxicated, death-seeking, isolationist . . ."

It's not easy living under the same roof with a Smith College education, if you're a man. My wife, who is better educated and smarter than I am, is telling me all this a few days later while standing in front of the mirror, naked, stabbing the air with her toothbrush, her breasts tremoring slightly with every thrust. I'm staring down past my slight paunch, so I don't have to look at Julie's face, watching my penis shrivel from some errant wintry draft. I'm having this weird out-of-body feeling again, except this time instead of being dead I am stuck in some installation put on at the Whitney Museum. *Adam & Eve Argument: Morning After the Expulsion.* I glance up for a moment to steal a look at Julie's face. On closer inspection, the foam at the corners of her mouth is only Tom's of Maine.

There are moments in a relationship when you feel that you are not just individuals trying to solve a personal problem, but representatives of your gender, acting out some social drama. Over Julie's shoulder I see a chorus of angry women, between the ages of thirty and forty, hundreds of thousands strong, all being channeled through my wife.

I can't quite make out everything they are saying, but I sure know what it means: revolution.

After decades of trying to get to the promised land, women have finally figured out that success, as defined by men, is not necessarily what they bargained for. Never mind pay parity and glass ceilings—the dirty little secret that women have discovered is that the world of male work is a temple full of false gods. Its treacherous theology works like this: After years of killing yourself to get to the top of the pyramid, you arrive, expecting to find the celestial executive dining room, only to have your heart ripped out and eaten and the smoking hulk of your body tossed over the edge to be cannibalized by those coming after you. Yes, it's perverse, but for some reason men find pleasure in it.

Women, of course, have the option of having better things to do—like perpetuating the species, for instance. But here the problem becomes more complex. Our particular point in gender history comes equipped with a "Catch–22" quandary for women. Choose Option #1: Exercise the biological imperative, abandon your job, go back to "being a mother," and you lose social status, income, and maybe your career. Choose Option #2: place career over biology, and you become a bit of a freak, acquire stigma, lose social status, and forfeit biological and spiritual fulfillment.

That leaves Option #3. Take the Great Leap Forward. Do both career and kids. The risk for a woman is huge, and what every woman wants to know, as long as she's throwing dice at the big table, is: What is my man going to do? Is he going to stand by me? Is he going to discard his centuries-old ways and become a full partner in raising a family? Or is he going to cling to the skirts of his ancient prerogatives and leave me holding the bag?

Welcome to the new primal scene. Eve with ovu-kit in one hand and cellular in the other. And Adam? All I can say about the new Adam is that I'm still feeling pretty primitive. I'm look-ing over my own shoulder for support and see nothing. Where is the gathering of sages, the accumulated male wisdom of the ages, or at least of the last three decades? Where is my band of brothers, my support system to help explain what I'm feeling, to breathe verbal life into the inner mud of my emotions? For the moment, the men's point of view is somewhere else, huddled in a sweat lodge muttering Amerindian mantras, or boarding a bus for a march, or gathering in intimate groups of, say, 60,000 in some stadium to listen to some Billy Graham wannabe and bad choir music.

Right now, I don't have a clue other than recognizing that to face one of life's most meaningful moments as a complete cipher is, to say the least, disappointing. Having done what I needed to do to get us pregnant, what now? Now, when I feel shriveled and impotent in the face of change.

Things were so much easier before the miscarriage, ten months ago. We had made a mutual decision to go for it, and Julie went off the pill. It's not that we didn't think about becoming parents. The secret was that it happened so fast that we didn't have *too* much time to think. Judging from the experience of most of our friends, we anticipated at least a six months' grace period or preamble before we had to deal with the actual reality of parenthood.

In the beginning, we kept it light. Our sex life, like that of so many other married couples, had become fat and lazy over the years. Going off the pill brought sex back to the level of being a teenager again—or maybe in our mid-twenties. Sex was no longer about relationship maintenance, or conflict resolution, or stress reduction. It was just fun.

The apparatus we'd been carrying between our legs for the last four decades worked perfectly. Almost exactly one month after she stopped taking the pill, Julie missed her first period. Several days later, we were dancing around our first positive pregnancy test.

We were amazed that everything seemed to work so smoothly. Easily 50 percent of our friends and acquaintances who are trying to have babies have had infertility problems. Paul and Astrid across the street, who are in their early thirties, have been trying for two years and are just beginning to see a reproductive endocrinologist. Joseph and Joan were in an IVF program, Joan having a serious case of endometriosis. My best friend Gary and his wife, Louise, went through a radically new IVF procedure, because Gary's vas deferens—the tube connecting his testicles to his prostate—is missing, and Louise has ovarian cysts. Jonathan and Carey have given up on IVF altogether and are trying to adopt.

Those first few days—it was as if someone had passed a magic wand over our lives. We were transported on hopes we never knew we had. We were always giddy about something. We put aside our postmodern irony and held hands at the slightest provocation; called each other repeatedly when apart; beheld each other with bliss-glazed eyes as often as we could; and noted with rapture, for the first time in our lives, passing children. The silliness crested on a ride up to my parents' house for Easter, as we spent two hours in the car verbally riffing and riffling through our respective wish books of names. Amid the backscreen projection of Route 17's New Jersey shopping malls and rural New York convenience stores, we tested the ear- and mouth-feel of Amelia and Amanda, Olivia and Eden, Tristan and Julian, Samuel and Roland.

Then the wand passed over us again. Easter Sunday found us in a panic, leaving a message with our OB/GYN's service at 4 A.M. I had stirred awake to find Julie weeping quietly. Some cramps that she had felt earlier had become steadily worse. Julie had been spotting occasionally, ever since her missed period; but since spotting is not abnormal, and since it had quieted down recently, we had begun to think that the pregnancy was sticking. The Big M was, of course, what we were worried about, but I was also afraid of an ectopic pregnancy, an extremely painful and medically serious condition where the fertilized egg implants in the Fallopian tube, growing until it ruptures the tube.

It felt surreal to be sitting up in bed in a farmhouse in upstate New York waiting for our Upper East Side OB/GYN to call; but call she did, within five minutes. To her undying credit, at 4 A.M. on Easter morning, Dr. Ann Spyros was unruffled and reassuring. She told us not to worry, that it was too early for an ectopic pregnancy, and to see her as soon as we returned to New York City. Several days later Julie came back from the appointment. She was fine, but the pregnancy was gone. We were to wait for two months before trying again, enough time for Julie to have another period and make sure her ovaries and uterus were functioning properly.

One small problem: We were spooked. It didn't matter that Spyros had reassured us that miscarriages were normal, and that almost all women, many without realizing it, had at least one miscarriage experience. It didn't matter that the books said that miscarriages were actually positive, indicating something profoundly wrong with the developing embryo. It didn't matter that my mother—who had generally kept her distance from Julie— had confided to us in a rare moment of bonding that she had had five miscarriages on the way to having five kids, which I guess made me a fifty-fifty proposition.

What followed was limbo. Life-decision-making paralysis (there is no doubt some German compound term for this state). We both took it differently. For Julie, the reaction to the miscarriage took the form of an argument with her body. She felt betrayed; a thirty-seven-year dialog had all of a sudden become tenuous and contentious.

For me, the impact was more subtle, more symbolic, and ultimately more debilitating. On the outside, I was the Man of Science. Since part of what I do professionally is health science documentaries for television, and consulting for the medical industry, including a major academic fertility center, I actually know something about the female anatomy other than what has been passed on to me through locker rooms, pornography, and personal inspection. I was reassuring. I told her to see the miscarriage as a trial run. See it, Julie, I said, not as failure, but as proof that the amazingly complex organic Rube Goldberg mechanism you've been carrying around all these years actually works. Above all, I said, do not attach symbolic importance to the miscarriage. This is not about the mind, but about the body, and your body is perfectly normal. Let's not overdetermine the situation. Let's not freight a biological event with superstition and mythology. Let's keep it as light as possible. Let's just keep going forward, as if nothing happened, and try again at the appropriate moment. Let's just get on with it.

Meanwhile, it was I who was loading the dice of meaning. Two months later, the first appropriate moment came and went. Three months—another opportunity passed. It seemed that whenever the four- to five-day window of fertility appeared, I was mysteriously absent. I pleaded exhaustion. I worked late, and came to bed after Julie had gone to sleep. I scheduled late dinner dates. I drank too much. I picked fights. Whatever it was, I always made sure it was too late for sex.

Finally, Julie called me on it. What could I say? I said a lot of things. I said a lot of nothing.

I still don't know for sure what I was going through emotionally. There are plenty of words to describe emotional states—anguish, euphoria—but not many related to the absence of emotion, except for that catch-all "depression," or those fancier French terms like "ennui" or "anomie." This was more like your cable TV going off-line for several weeks, leaving you switching between eighty channels of static and snow, occasionally punctuated by an electronic hiccup and the flash of some random, scrambled image from your past.

What had started out as a semi-impulsive leap of faith, something akin to "it just feels right," had reverted to an attempt to make a rational decision. It finally reached the point where we actually found ourselves scheduling appointments with each other to talk about why we should have kids. When we compared notes, it turned out that we held many of our doubts in common.

After a couple of these bruising sessions, we were finally able to identify and actually voice our fears. We felt that having children put everything we held dear—our ambitions, our relationship, our emotional life, and yes, our lifestyle—at risk.

Having turned the corner on my mid-thirties, I had only recently felt that my life had caught up with my body and was living in it. I had spent much of this time getting over the hangover created during my protracted adolescence. Now, my writing career had finally begun to accelerate. After surviving the first four tumultuous years of marriage, our relationship had begun to find a livable rhythm in the last two (albeit with occasional doses of couple therapy). We also had money, for a change.

Having children seemed like acquiring a potential pathology. I mean, why change? That's a valid question, isn't it? I had already suffered, struggled, and achieved what I thought was a considerable measure of material and spiritual happiness. Where is the rationality in trading in the happiness one has achieved for an undeniably difficult and painful process that holds out the possibility of great reward, but also great failure? Yes, one hears, incessantly, that having children is an irreplaceable feeling, conjures a love supreme, and offers an experience whose profundity dwarfs all others. However, these platitudes—usually offered by sleep-deprived, zombie-parents to whom you want to say "Have you looked in the mirror lately, bud?" or by your own parents, whose credibility rating is automatically zero—butt up against the painful reality that many of us carry within. What happens if you didn't particularly like yourself as a child?

Take me, for example. I was a fat, noisy, hyperactive child, who went on to become a slimmer, noisy, hyperactive adolescent with a bad body image—a juggernaut of fantastical ideas and directionlessness, who on the first try failed most of society's tests, including my first try at college. Okay, so most people have baggage; but in my own mind, there was a permanent platoon of redcaps following me around.

I had already survived myself once. Why would I want to recapitulate the experience?

Nor did I particularly like other people's children. In an era of "family values" I was W. C. Fields reincarnate. Children were willful, impossible to control, and intrusive, and invariably grew up into disappointing adolescents who were monsters of insecurity and self-loathing, who expressed themselves by hating their parents.

Nor did I particularly like parents of children as a group. On the whole, they seemed like a beaten, unspontaneous lot, perpetually huddled in little groups, bunkered into their houses, neurotic with worry, obsessed with ludicrous minutiae, and worst of all, unwelcome in movie theaters and finer restaurants. My buddies who had joined this dubious club seemed suddenly neutered and gelded by practicality. Parents seemed to me to be people who had run out of ideas, people who had turned to biology when their ideals and goals had eluded them.

When I learned to have goals, being a father was not one of them. I wanted and needed to be a writer. This, of course, meant a life of greater than normal risk—potentially a lifetime of trying without guarantee of reward. To this end, I had conformed most of my life choices. I chose Julie as my partner, the only woman I had ever met who was willing to support me with heart, soul, and at times pocketbook, and, almost as important, had parents that accepted me—most other prospective in-laws were ready to call the police when they found out I had no intention of joining the corporate workforce. I was also willing to pay my dues, working my way up from the proverbial mailroom to writing press releases and every other conceivable variety of copy, while I continued to work on poems, short stories, and novels.

So I had already chosen my big risk in life. Taking on anything more seemed like sheer folly—like shooting craps and playing poker simultaneously.

To my credit, there was also a part of me that was willing to concede that all this was an elaborate argument for self-absorption, if not self-delusion. Was I so arrogant that I thought I was already complete? Did I not understand how profound the experience of having children could be? Could I afford not to deepen myself as a human being?

So, whether in serious conversation on sofas, or in yelling matches conducted naked in front of mirrors, this was the ball of hopelessly tangled string, the Gordian knot of worries that had replaced my brain. Try as I might, I could not undo it with reason, or slice through it with will.

Luckily, Julie could.

• • •

Park Slope, Brooklyn, is an idyllic place to have children. There is plenty of work, money, resources, child care, and community. As a group of expectant parents, we would seem blessed. Yet listening to us worry about money, career, relationships, and birth defects, you would never know that we have more wealth, more education, more information, more technology, more health care, more kitchen appliances—more of everything than any other group at any other time in history. What is the problem? Where is all this anxiety coming from?

I think we suffer from what the Renaissance Italians called "horror vacui," the fear of empty space. It refers to a condition in mural painting where every available square inch of space has been filled with something, usually something decorative and meaningless. Today, we have become information obsessed. We insist on filling up all empty space in our brains with data. As with painting, the addition of too many elements flattens out reality. We lose perspective, and the human dimension and its themes are diminished. We suffer from our self-inflicted riches. We compulsively keep our lives so full that there is no silence left to nourish us. Nowhere is this obsession more apparent than the need to fill the biggest space of all, the future.

Men, in particular, seem to suffer when they make decisions about the future, especially about becoming fathers. I asked my friend Sandy Robertson, M.D., what he thought.

Why are men so fucked up, Sandy?
Our cortex is the storytelling part of our brain. Strategic, future-oriented, past-oriented. It has the capacity to do abstract operations, and because of this, we end up, around eleven years old, capable of suffering from existential anxiety.

"Oh, my God, what about the future, especially given my past?" So, we have something that as far as we can tell, no other living creature has: anxiety about an unknown future, made complex by our capacity to remember our past in more than an instinctual or primitive way. It is our blessing, and our curse.

Sandy thinks the problem lies in the stories we tell ourselves. Sandy is not your average shrink. He is a shrink on steroids, a psychiatrist with specialties in neurology and child psychiatry, who has studied with Tibetan and Zen Buddhists, and who has a new way of thinking about the mind.

I got to know Sandy through our friends Vera and Hideo. They have two children, one from Hideo's first marriage and one together. Hideo is a very successful painter with an international reputation. Vera is from a wealthy English family. When Vera became pregnant again, Hideo bugged. They went to see Sandy so that Hideo could get a tune-up.

"One of the things that I come across often in my practice are men in great anxiety about becoming fathers for the first time, or again. The suffering that they do, the worrying about the first child or another child are based on their wishes to stay in control of their current life circumstances.

"One man said, 'I've just got my life where I want it. My wife and I are really happy together. A child, I'm afraid, would really spoil everything, and throw in disarray that which I've worked so hard to attain.'

"The same irrational projection can hold true with having additional children. Another said: 'We've finally gotten enough room for the four of us. Now that we're pregnant again, how can we possible manage? We don't have enough money to build another room, we can't afford to move again, I'm not going to get another raise for five years, blah, blah, blah' . . . All the suffering begins to show up.

"Peasants in Mexico don't think like this. Pregnant! Happy! Celebrate! Another baby? We'll have four sleeping in our bed instead of three. We'll feed them. We'll work harder. We'll make more tortillas. They have a very different attitude about life. Children are treasures."

So, are stories of control actually stories of suffering in disguise?

Generating anxiety based on irrational projections of the future—I define this as suffering. Irrational fear of pain in the future, leading to the physiological fight-flight response in the body, producing an avoidance action. When you are pregnant or thinking about pregnancy, anxiety about controlling the situation is the wrong conversation. It's a story that creates fear, because there is no control. I counsel my patients that we are never in control of anything, ever. The best we can do is manage in the here and now.

As I leave Sandy, I can't help thinking about his Mexican peasants. My mind flashed back to the fertility center where I consult. We had made a big push to reach out to the Hispanic community, to override their religious and cultural inhibitions and resistance to what we in the trade call ARTS, or "assisted reproductive technologies." The fruit of our efforts sat in the waiting room, a working-class couple, Ray and Islin Ramirez.

I couldn't help thinking that all the technology and knowledge that waited for them beyond the inevitable double doors and the nurses' station only pointed out a greater historical irony, and perhaps the widening gulf between the biological truths of our bodies and the stories we can tell. Once upon a time, having children, reproducing, was probably the first encounter that man had with mass production, the mass production that nature requires. Everything else—books, spears, bowls, clothing, shoes, perhaps even ideas—they all had to be made, painstakingly, one at a time. Children could be made easily, and by the laws of mortality, needed to be made in abundance.

Now the tables have turned. The rest of reality is mass-produced, but our children? We make them one at a time, and they have to be perfect. All the couples in the waiting room, and the rest of us beyond it, have become artisans, refining our art until one sperm can be guided to one egg, one child made to fit one cushioned slot in our lives.

My theory is that we have all become afraid of making something. Imagine if the technology, the appliances, the trappings, the conveniences we have gathered around us are an expression, not of a search for knowledge, but instead, of our unease. Imagine if what we think of as tools are not tools at all, but restraints of a sort, to help us stay where we are.

The more control we are given, the less control we have. The closer we come to being gods, it would seem, the more we suffer.

In the beginning there was the word, and that word was . . . ambivalence.

To be fair, we are not the only ones with a cosmic case of performance anxiety. If we have difficulty in facing the conflicts in our own individual creation stories, we can take some comfort in the knowledge that what we feel is an ancient anxiety that all cultures have felt over the forces that are unleashed when we create life and the difficulty involved in controlling those forces.

Most creation stories carry within them the seeds of ambivalence about creation. Look at our own Judeo-Christian story. It has a God who broods over the void, creates evil as well as good, witnesses murder in the second generation, and then decides to start all over again by flooding the world and wiping the slate practically clean.

It's no wonder that human beings feel insecure about entering the metaphysical fray, as we do when we create life.

MONTH TWO

LA NAUSEA

My favorite joke when friends ask how things are going is: "Julie is pregnant, but I'm the one who's doing all the throwing up."

I have two images of Julie. One is of her sitting in a chair, doubled over, waiting to throw up. The second, Julie sitting in a chair, doubled over, waiting to throw up, but meanwhile talking on the telephone. I've been watching and half-listening to Julie talk on the telephone for what seems like a week straight. News spreads fast, especially if you're working the phones nonstop. I never realized that she had so many friends. Or maybe they're not actually friends at all. Maybe she's run out of friends and is calling complete strangers at random. "You don't know me, but my name is Julie, and I'm going to be a mother!" Today, all of the New York metro area; tomorrow, the entire Eastern Seaboard will know.

What is there to talk about at this point? As far as I can tell, it's mostly about *what is going to happen to Julie's body*.

I can imagine them on the other end of the phone line, their myriad faces reflexively screwed up into masks of concern, saying things like: "Do you feel nauseous?" "How often are you urinating?" "Have you gained any weight yet?" "Do your breasts hurt?" "Are you constipated?"

And then there are particularly eye- and hair-raising responses from Julie, like: "So your husband had trouble with your vaginal discharge in the sixth month?"

I'm trying to think about what I can compare it to in my own experience. For example, I'm trying to remember the last time I had a long conversation with a buddy about my penis, or the sensitivity of my nipples, or how my prostate feels a little tender when I pee, or how I had an unusually large and satisfying, corkscrew-shaped bowel movement this morning.

Women love talking about their bodies. This is what ultimately got us pregnant in the first place. Julie's way of cutting through our ambivalence was to listen to her friends, most of whom were breeding at the time. She would return from a baby shower, or from a visit to a friend with a newborn, or put down the telephone after talking to Alice in Boston about the trials of putting her three-year-old to bed, or look up from a six-page, single-spaced letter from her friend Lauren, describing the adventures of a swashbuckling childbirth in a field hospital located somewhere in southern Africa—two days of back labor, awash in blood, urine, and feces in a facility without anesthesia—and there would be this expression, as she looked around the dwelling of our life, that there was something important missing, as if we were in danger of losing our animation and becoming the spiritual equivalents of furniture. My Husband, the Armchair.

Her desire to have a baby scared the shit out of me, but what other choice did I have? What right did I have—a person whose sole approach to decision making rests on the outcome of competing doubts—to stand in the way of another who shows the slightest preference based on the merest sliver of certainty? Even if that certainty comes from instinct or intuition rather than reasoning? After all, were we really meant to *think* about reproduction?

If nature depended on humans, men in particular, to rationalize having children, we would never have made it as a species. Can you imagine Mr. Australopithecus doing the numbers, weighing the cost/benefit of reproduction? "Let's see. Today, I have to go out and trot twenty miles around the savanna with my buddies in search of food, put down a few mastodons, risking major orthopedic trauma if not death, then schlep back all the meat, protecting it from marauding Neanderthals, and get back to base camp in time to give Austro Junior a bath, read to him from some favorite hunter-gatherer stories, and then put him to sleep?" Or better yet, "How am I going to become the best cave painter in the valley if I have to be a father, too?" I think not.

So nature, in all her wisdom, invented desire.

I'm beginning to realize that there may be some jealousy operating here. Julie's ability to call up friends and talk is leaving me feeling a little left out. As an experiment, I spend some time reaching out to my buddies, trying to create the same effect.

"You'll never sleep again." —Andy, who seems to get plenty of sleep, most of it on his feet.

"You'll never have a moment to yourself again." —Joseph, who would prefer to spend his whole life in a room by himself.

"You'll never go to the movies, or go out to dinner again." —Mark, whose idea of a good time is to travel far to find bad Greek food, when he can get it around the corner.

"You'll never have sex again." —Charles, who's so out of it after the arrival of his second child that I can see why no one, including his wife, would want to have sex with him.

"You'll never have sex again, but a baby is an incredible Babe Magnet." —Theo, who never gives up.

After several more attempts to draw upon the support and collective wisdom of my circle of male intimates, I've come to the conclusion that what I really need is new friends.

Life is pretty much normal except for the fact that I have a prospective barfing wife on my hands. I'm trying to camouflage it as best I can, but emotionally, I'm not responding too well. I think the problem here is that Julie isn't actually *throwing up*, just threatening.

We'll be walking through a restaurant and Julie will slow down and signal me with that peculiar look of dread and anticipation. Always vigilant, I quickly steer her into the ladies' room, shooing away a covey of women anxious to pee. Then, after watching her stare into a toilet for several minutes with a faraway look that promises the vomiting of galaxies . . . nothing.

Or we'll wake up in the morning and instead of the usual kiss or snuggle, she'll look at me and say, "Can you get a bucket?" I'll pop out of bed and sprint to the garden shed next to the kitchen to retrieve a pail, and race back to her as if I'm carrying news from Marathon, only to have her lean over it and moan for a while, with an occasional cough, or hack, or dry heave with some spittle, as a promise of things to come. But never the actual main event. I've done this now for two consecutive weeks, and I just can't get any relief.

Finally someone gives us an invaluable piece of advice. Crackers. Not Ritz, not Wheat Thins, not Carr's Water Biscuits, just plain saltines. It works brilliantly, except for one little thing. Everywhere we go, everywhere we live—crumbs.

•   •   •

It is the middle of the day and Julie is lying on our bed sleeping. I am perched on the side of the bed watching her belly, which rises and settles tidelike with her breath. Her sleep is infectious, and as I look down at her belly, it is as if I am viewing a face through water. A moment later, her belly smiles at me as I drift off.

She has been very tired lately, and pale. For her to be napping in the middle of the day is abnormal and disturbing. She usually finds it impossible to nap, and she's a workaholic. Her habits now seemed more defined by sleep than by waking. She moves between islands of sleep. Even her wakefulness appears to be a form of animated sleep, her movements turning heavy and deliberate as if she were feeling her way through the hormonal fog of her changing physiology.

Things are changing. Time and meaning are snapping their moorings. Daily objects and events become part of something else. Julie's body is no longer Julie's body. It's the vessel, the pod, the hull, the hive, the chrysalis, and every other loopy simile that my mind can concoct. Of course, this amount of meaning can't possibly stay put. It moves around. It overflows into every other part of your life. I can no longer just go into my kitchen—which is my favorite place, because I like to cook—because that's where food for the Vessel is being prepared. Or I can never just go into the bathroom to take a shit, because that's where the Local Manifestation of the Eternal Feminine bathes. Or I can't just flop down on my couch to finish reading the *Times* because maybe I should be doing something for the Bearer of the Eight Cells That Are My Child, if only I could figure out what to do.

Sometimes, I can't decide whether I'm losing my mind, or whether I've watched too many reruns of *The Prisoner*. I'm Patrick McGoohan. I'm running down the street of this quaint British seaside town, which really isn't a seaside town at all but Brooklyn in disguise. There are children everywhere, holding red balloons, following me with their eyes. Oh, God, who's that in the bookstore? It's Julie, buying a copy of *What to Expect When You're Expecting*. Who's that in the clothing store? It's Julie buying XXL underwear with spandex inserts capable of stretching to infinity. I run screaming home for shelter, only to see the walls of my bedroom peel back, exposing a control room full of sinister-looking scientists and bureaucrats. Everything I've thought of up to now as nature is actually the manipulations of an obscure British government agency that has taken over Julie's body to launch a global conspiracy called Change.

That's on a good day. On a bad day it gets much worse.

Like Roquentin in Sartre's *La Nausée*, I feel unplugged from meaning. I go about my daily activities, but the weight and substance seem to be draining from the intentions behind my actions and movements. I could do something, or I could not do it: It really doesn't seem to matter. As the idea of Julie's belly grows larger—I say idea as I can detect no actual change yet, even after numerous surprise inspections—I'm beginning to feel like one of those figures from newsreels dangling from the dirigible's mooring line, legs churning in the air like a doomed terrier.

And somehow the tempo has shifted behind the scenes and behind my thoughts. As if one moment I was imagining myself standing on a bar table leading the crowd in a round of "Danny Boy," or on stage with Aerosmith playing air guitar, only to turn around and find myself in a orchestra pit with the ghost of Von Karajan staring me down, waiting for me to come to my senses so that the production of *Götterdämmerung* can continue.

Men don't really live in their bodies—that's the reason I'm having so many out-of-body experiences. We live in our stories. But the problem with men's stories, besides the fact that they go on forever, is that they are built without a sense of actual time. For men, time is a fiction: a convenience ("I really don't have the time to do that, honey"), a stratagem ("If there were but world enough and time, dear lady," etcetera), and at best an artifice called the future, where things like emotions and memories are stored for that day when we actually have the time to experience them. Only when our body's reality starts to intrude upon our stories do we give time its due by throwing a fit we call a mid-life crisis. Men, ultimately, would like to live outside time, but time is what structures reality, and that is why men live with women.

Women carry time in their bodies. We acknowledge this by calling it a "biological clock," but give it a negative connotation of a limitation. A positive way would be to look at a woman's body as a kind of biological metronome, referenced to rhythms more fundamental than the insane chronometers of productivity and advertising; a botanical filter or lens that upon maturing focuses the different story lines of a relationship, and fuses the fictions of men and women into the reality of family and children.

For some, the female botanical metaphor is all-defining. For the Tangilka of Papua, New Guinea, women are at the center of a botanical concept of growth. The mother is the base of the family tree; her children are cuttings or transplants. When a girl is given in marriage, the family of her husband receives the bounty of a "cutting" from the maternal base.

In time's rainforest, women are the trees, and men are the preening and warbling birds, living and dying in their canopies. For me, the structure of Julie's habits and desires have always been the house in which I've lived. I have come to accept this, and I think it is also true for many of the men I know, although they may not be capable of admitting it. We live in an age when it is easy for men to be confused about what is demanded of us, because most of the cultural scripts are obsolete or missing. Today, life demands daily adaptations, daily strategies, daily teamwork, and daily faith. Faced with this, men have had to come home to compose their lives.

Books form a skyline on Julie's bedside table. They have titles like *What to Expect When You're Expecting, The Well Pregnancy Book, Active Birth,* and *The Birth Partner.* (Hmm ... wonder who that is?) These tomes look scary to me and, frankly, I've been doing my best to ignore their arrival. Each looks weighty enough to stop an oncoming bus. Scariest of all, one of these books is in Italian—*Il Grande Libro del Bambino*—a language that, last time I checked, neither of us speak.

Julie has become totally absorbed. It seems as if no matter from what viewing angle or time of day, one of these books has replaced her head. My favorite is when we're both lying in bed. I'm poring over the latest computer catalog or *New York* magazine. Occasionally I sneak a glance Julie's way. I see a birth manual with an unbelievably bad piece of cover art wavering on a stalk that used to be Julie's neck. Her left hand, moving autonomically to a box of saltines, is a train of soldier ants carrying an endless succession of crackers to her mandibles. Occasionally a shower of fine wheat dust interrupts the relentless crunching to fall like dry snow onto her nightgown.

Days pass and the inevitable happens. Mysteriously the birth manuals seem to be pursuing some ancient migratory route and begin appearing on my bedside table. I ignore them for a week, until a light coating of dust forms on their jackets. Through our nightly reading rituals, I can tell that Julie is watching me for any signs of self-initiated interest. I feel like a subject in a Jane Goodall experiment:

Chubby ignored the books for several days, until one day the most amazing thing happened. He picked one up, and realizing it was about the female primate reproductive experience, immediately acquired an apprehension of language and read voraciously to the point of overstimulation. We subsequently had to sedate him to save his life.

Finally, being able to take a hint as well as any man, and feeling as if my bedside collection of computer magazines was in danger of being burned, I relent. One night in full view of the Pregnancy Police, I throw down *Geek World* with a show of disgust and pick up the nearest pregnancy tome with gusto worthy of the Cultural Revolution.

The first riddle I solve is the provenance of *Il Grande Libro del Bambino*. An inscription on the frontispiece is from our neighbor Cecilia, who is Italian. Likewise, many of the rest of the books have also traveled from the four corners. Another inscription reads from Maureen, Kotzebue, Alaska. Still another from Lauren, this time from the northernmost reaches of Scotland. I realize that each of these books has helped guide the birth of at least one child into the world, if not many more, judging from the dog-eared pages, and that Julie's friends had passed them along as soon as they heard she was pregnant.

The sweetness of these inscriptions and the gestures behind them are no match for the shock I feel when I actually start leafing through the pages. One book opens with a photo essay of a birth. A woman is lying on her back, naked, on a bed. At the beginning, her face is a half-smile. Her huge, slack breasts are beached jellyfish on the pendulous sphere of her stomach. Below her stomach is a large, black, hairy, algae bloom that I presume is her vagina. In subsequent frames her face contorts into a sequence of grimaces that I can only imagine signify unimaginable pain. Finally, something resembling a human-shaped muskrat emerges. In the last scene, a man with an ugly shirt and a bad haircut appears, as well as the inscription, ". . . not only a new baby is born, but a new family too." The whole thing looks like it was shot through a mud puddle.

I quickly move on to another book. This one is filled with black-and-white pictures of women giving birth in various squatting positions. Again, their faces are howling with pain, and many of them are supported by half-naked men with more bad haircuts, who I assume are their husbands. Most are also attended by other women who appear to be nurses or midwives, who kneel by the women's vaginas with the same expectant pose that I use when I'm operating a vending machine. It all seems so alien to me, in defiance of everything I have ever seen or learned from television. To top off its bad-dream status, the quality of the photographs is horrible, on a par with classic, early pornography.

The mystery of the quality of the photographs and the haircuts is solved when I check the copyright on the two books. Both were produced in the late seventies in England. A quick skim of their introductions reveals loud rants against the medical system as well as a call to arms for women's rights and natural childbirth.

All I can think of at this point is: "If this is natural childbirth, maybe we should check out some books with titles like *The Unnatural Childbirth,* or *Five Easy Steps to Immaculate Conception and Delivery.*" This is not what I imagined, although in all candor I can't say anything comes to mind when I try to imagine what it's going to be like when Julie gives birth. I know this sounds ridiculous—after all, I've written health science documentaries and consulted with medical schools—but the part where Julie gives birth is a complete blank. I can't imagine Julie looking anything like those squatting, disheveled, pendulous creatures, and I certainly can't imagine myself in the place of those guys. I have great hair.

Next I pick up *What to Expect When You're Expecting*. Written and published in the United States in the mid-eighties, it gives you the Disney version of birth: clean, well-organized, well-written, and devoid of mystical allusions and pictures of multibreasted fertility goddesses taken from archeological dig sites. The figures giving birth, of which there are only two, are done in perfectly sensible and pedestrian pencil drawings. Best of all, the husband helping the woman in one of the illustrations has a hairdo like Race Bannon in Johnny Quest. Now this is something I can handle.

Suddenly, I develop a curiosity about whether it has a section on the men's experience. Flipping to the book's index, I search under the M's, but find no "Men" between "Membranes" and "Menstruation," nor anything under "Male" between "Making love" and "Mastitis." Nor do I find "Husband" between "Human chorionic gonadotropin" and "Hyperventilation." More than a little disappointed, what I do find, finally, is a section called "Last But Not Least," with a subsection titled, "Fathers Are Expectant Too."

Last but not least? Whom are they trying to kid? What is last, if not least? The men's section follows a chapter describing the first six weeks of the postpartum experience. And another thing: I find it strange that men are referred to as fathers before they are technically fathers. I certainly don't think of myself as a father yet. Ironic, don't you think, considering that a cornerstone of the feminist movement is definitely not to consider a woman a mother until the fetus becomes a newborn. Finally, the fucking section is 10 pages long in a book with 351 pages. Is someone trying to send me a message here? If I were to treat this as an analogy, it would mean that the man's experience is valued at roughly 2.85 percent of the pregnancy experience as a whole. That means that out of the 280-

day, 40-week pregnancy period, I would only have to be involved for eight days. While this might literally describe the state of circumstances in many marriages, somehow, judging from Julie's intentions, I don't think that's going to fly in my case.

The text is workmanlike, straightforward, and earnest, and is basically a quick shopping list of seemingly obvious worries: fear of sex; anxiety over your wife's health; anxiety over your baby's health; anxiety over your wife's looks; anxiety about passing out during the labor and delivery; and so on. The net effect is both unintentionally humorous and irritating. I can't quite pinpoint what bothers me about the whole effort, except why they bothered. For one thing, there are several flaws in strategy and design. Most men that I know do not respond well to being told that they are going to feel afraid or nervous, even when that is a foregone conclusion.

Then, there seems to be some central rallying point missing that's appealing to the male ego: some effective metaphor, some edifying context. For example, a short section with the heading "Get an Education" encourages men to read everything they can get their hands on about pregnancy, but doesn't provide a compelling purpose. What's the point? What is the man supposed to do with this information?

The problem here is that the whole attitude of this book mirrors the attitude of society. The chapter's first paragraph pays lip service to the man as the "equal partner-in-reproduction," but then condescendingly implies that the man's practical role is nonexistent. I'm sorry, but you don't have to be well-educated to be a hand holder or a blocking dummy. Then the rest of the chapter proceeds to deal almost exclusively with the feelings of alienation men will feel because of this condition, rather than concentrating on strategies and reasons that a man might actually be useful. It seems to me to be a self-fulfilling prophecy. Granted that the book is meant primarily for women; however, to refer to a man as some sort of passive object, or even a victim, is not to get his attention.

There's also this really weird section on sympathetic pregnancy, which surprisingly takes up a whole page (10 percent of the proceedings). It says that anywhere from 11 to 65 percent of men mimic their wives' pregnancy with symptoms including "abdominal pain, appetite changes, weight gain, food cravings, constipation, leg cramps, dizziness, fatigue, mood swings, and nausea and vomiting."

This is much more than I can stomach.

There is something I need to know that no pregnancy manual can possibly tell me: What is going to happen now that Julie has stopped taking her antidepressants?

Part of me can't help but recognize the irony, perhaps even the absurdity of this worry. How indulgent. But the good soldier, the grunt who lives out every day in the foxhole of the marital quotidian and has lived to tell the tale, knows how important this is.

One of the things that I have always loved about my wife is her depths. My wife is a creature of history. While most of America comes with that polymerized "new car" smell and a plasticity of persona and attitude, she is Old World. She smells of pastries. Butter, cream, caramelized fruit, bitter chocolate—the Hotel Sacher in Vienna where her mother would go as a young child to eat sweets, before the family left, two years after the Anschluss.

This may sound crazy, but I think one of the things that brought us together is that both our mothers were refugees—my mother walked twenty miles a day during the Korean War, carrying one of my older brothers on her back and leading the other by the hand—and we both understand that there are things that even

America can't replace or heal; not in a generation, not in two. If most others seem to me stricken with contentlessness, Julie, like many other Jews, is burdened from having received more than her share of irreconcilable information. History can have an indelible effect on a family's mind, that peculiar creature born of the interaction of inherited narratives and biology.

I have all sorts of ideas about why Julie gets depressed, but in the end it is also an illness, a province of the body, and no amount of philosophy or understanding packs the punch of 100 milligrams of Wellbutrin. I can see the little pills beaming at me through their amber vial every time I walk into the bathroom. The layout of the logo makes each pill seem like a grinning Cyclops, a smiley face for the millennium. But I bear no illusions. What I mostly feel is gratitude. Without our little friends to tip the serotonin balance in our favor, our little world would lose its delicate equilibrium and hurl itself to pieces.

And now that we have to do without them for at least the next nine months? All I can say is that I feel as vulnerable as she must feel. And I will be watching her, lovingly and carefully.

This morning I crawled to the kitchen to make my usual morning coffee. Illy Café espresso, two teaspoons of sugar, a healthy dollop of half-and-half: a caffeine, sugar, and fat cocktail better known as Rocket Fuel.

Morning coffee has become a solitary ritual. Julie sleeps later than usual these days, and besides, has developed an aversion to the smell of coffee. She thought it would be the hardest thing to give up—because of the caffeine—but at the moment, she can't even stand being in the same room.

Five minutes after I finish, I start to gag—a sort of dry hack at the back of the throat. This has become more and more common over the last month, and it's really irritating because it lasts long enough to make the rest of my morning ablutions difficult, like brushing my teeth and breathing at the same time. It's getting bad enough that I figure I'm beginning to develop an allergy to coffee, which is odd, because I've drunk coffee for twenty years now without incident. With breathtaking, java-junkie logic, I've begun to compensate by taking a prescription antihistamine. (Nothing like innovative measures to continue ingesting something you believe is poisoning you.)

The first attack passes. I make my move toward the bathroom, when I get a second, much more violent attack. Feeling my esophagus start to quake, I make it into the bathroom just in time to projectile vomit a jet of hot, brown liquid into the bathtub. I look at it, stunned with disbelief, as it starts to stream toward the drain. The smell of curdled half-and-half mixed with bile fills the morning air.

Okay, so maybe it's time to switch to herbal tea.

MONTH THREE

OF CATSHIT AND PARANOIA

The eradication of catshit is my life.

Every morning since Julie has known she was pregnant, it has been the same. Before my morning cup, before my shower, before my own ablutions, I strap on a thick pair of blue rubber gloves and clean out the cat pan. The little turds swim before my still-blurry eyes like fat worms on their desert island home. Somewhere in the background of my brain, the theme to *Gilligan's Island* is playing. A quick poke with my scooper and I've got the Skipper. A quick flick, and it's the Millionaire and his Wife. Another, and it's the Professor and Mary Ann. Funny, I can't find Gilligan this morning. Too bad: He'll have to be hunted down and exterminated.

What I'm doing is mounting an all-out campaign against an unseen enemy, which in this case consists of microorganisms called *Toxoplasma gondii*. They are found in cat feces and raw meat. The disease they cause, toxoplasmosis, is a very mild infection that usually involves no more than a slight fever and swollen glands. Most who contract it get over it without treatment, and without knowing they've had it at all. Unless, of course, you are an unborn fetus. Then the possibility exists that you might suffer brain damage, malformation, or death.

As with most things that threaten pregnancies, the actual odds are very small. A high percentage of people with cats and/or people who eat raw or rare meat have developed immunity. Of the small number of pregnant women who haven't developed immunity and who are exposed and who actually develop the disease, 40 percent pass it on to their fetuses. Of this group, two-thirds of the fetuses who are exposed are unharmed.

But that's not what you focus on. What you focus on are the stories of a friend of a friend who knows a couple whose baby was born with a birth defect. And since in our case, Julie's test comes back negative, showing no previous infection (which I find amazing as we have four cats and frequently eat steak tartare), and since I am not a gambling man, I strap on my blue gloves and head to the cat pan every morning.

I attack my project with the zeal of the Inquisition. My attitude is childlike and my fervor driven by a medieval sense of imagination—I keep visualizing germs everywhere like an infestation of demons and a baby with two heads and the body of a slug being born—and I suspect it is this quality of imagination that has kept Hollywood in business all these years.

My administrations become ridiculous. After disposing of the feces by double-sealing them in two plastic bags, I then go to the sink to scrub off any stowaway *Toxoplasma gondii* that may have stolen onto the surface of my gloves. I hang the gloves in their usual place, which is from a hook over the sink area. I'm about to walk away with pride in a job well done, when I notice that a few drops of water are dribbling off the gloves onto the clean dishes and flatware drying in the dish rack directly below.

"Could I have just contaminated all those clean dishes?" squeaks my little brain. What if one or two or a whole platoon of the little devils have escaped my precautions? What if Julie eats off the supposedly clean dishes, gets infected, and gives birth to a monster?

My brain is vapor-locked with indecision. Part of me, the Majority Party, just wants to go on. Take a shower. Have some herbal tea. Read the newspaper. But the Minority Party, the Loyal Opposition, the Party of Rectitude and Ought, keeps mentioning the unmentionable. Moments later I am rewashing all the dishes with quiet fury, thinking dark thoughts about the cats milling about my feet. They seem like nothing more than shit factories: mindless, four-legged earthworms plowing through yards of cat food, leaving ca-ca and disease in their wake. I have hellish fantasies about sewing up their rectums. Funny, I once thought of these same cats as my children.

Finally. Julie's midsection is starting to show. It started as an almost imperceptible thickening, and then it seems like I turned around one day and she'd swallowed a salad spinner. Julie is a tiny girl. If this is what she looks like at three months, she's going to resemble the Graf Zeppelin at six.

I'd like to say I feel relieved. After all, part of the problem has been a lack of physical evidence or, I should say, visual evidence, that what we're doing is for real and not some hysterical delusion. However, I also feel that denial is an overcriticized and underserved state of mind. Denial is a convenient fiction instituted by the cerebral cortex to counteract the constant invocation of the flight-fight response by the limbic system. In other words, denial is what allows you to stay calm and live your life. Physical change, however, while hardly making denial impossible, certainly makes it more difficult. Julie's ballooning stomach certainly relocates the pregnancy from the abstract to the concrete.

That strange sense of displacement I started feeling from the very beginning of the pregnancy, however, has not left; in fact, it has turned into a weird sense of isolation. How can I describe it? I remember an essay I read once by the feminist literary critic Julia Kristeva. I forget exactly which essay it was. The metaphor, however, I've never forgotten. Kristeva compares the pregnant woman to a Renaissance walled town. The wall of her abdomen, or uterus, is the protective barrier or perimeter that separates the world of her pregnancy from the outside world. And it is the internal world of the pregnancy to which she turns her attention and which she cultivates.

It is a remarkably beautiful image, and even more remarkable is that it's stuck by me all these years, considering that I read the essay in college, a time when having children was the furthest thing from my mind. Why this image, when I've forgotten everything I've ever read by the same author, and perhaps everything I've ever read from college, period?

It describes precisely how I feel. Julie is inside her "town." She's completely mobilized, busy making preparations. I mean this in the most literal way. She's already started buying baby clothes and furniture from the consignment shop on Carroll Street. She's already bought a baby seat and a backpack carrier. Every time she goes out now, no matter what the errand, she comes home with miniature T-shirts and jumpers. Occasionally she asks me with an irritating smile what I think of her purchases. What do I think? I think the baby is now about the size of a dragonfly nymph. How the fuck is it going to fit into that?

She's already rearranged the space in our apartment. What used to be my writing study will now be the baby's room. Meanwhile, baby supplies and clothing are streaming in. It seems that every other time I answer the door, it's UPS or Special Delivery with a parcel of baby clothes from California, or Scotland, or Alaska. Last week Simon, Julie's brother, and his wife, Mary, stopped by and left off a baby swing, a gift from her family in Hadley, Massachusetts—who, by the way, have never met us. There are literally bales of baby stuff stored in our upstairs closet and accumulating in our bedroom.

From my perspective, I am on the other side of that wall, wondering what is going on. Except it doesn't feel like a Renaissance town. The pace and urgency of the preparations feels more like that of the movie *When Worlds Collide*. That's the movie where an asteroid is going to destroy the Earth, and a select number of people have been chosen to leave on a rocket ship to colonize another planet. I suspect I'm not among the lucky ones.

It is not as if Julie were consciously ignoring me or abandoning me, but it does seem that she's drawn what she needs of the world inside her town, and left me on the outside. Inside, that's where the story is. Out here, there's no story. Out here, the world is void.

It started out with small, but irrepressible thoughts. Maybe it has something to do with the fact that Julie doesn't really walk anymore. She waddles. And when she goes out on errands or to meet with a client, I find myself thinking about her waddling, and I can't quite put down those thoughts. Maybe it's some ur-response from our Pleistocene ancestors. I mean Mr. Australopithecus takes one look at his mate waddling out of the cave and he's thinking: "Shit, there's no way she's going to be able to run from that big cat, or get out of the way of that charging mastodon." Me, I'm thinking the same thing: "There's no way Julie is going to be able to run from a mugger or sidestep that careening gypsy cab." Suddenly, I find myself tensing, crouching, getting ready to move, when the reality is that I'm in some boring business meeting or at my desk, and Julie's probably having tea with her girlfriends or quietly grazing at some shoe store.

Every day I take my paranoia to some new level. Just walking Julie around the neighborhood exhausts my awareness. Imagine yourself walking down the sidewalk with your pregnant wife, the story of your life playing through your mind. Between every crosswalk you're thinking that you don't really deserve this beautiful pregnancy, you're not worthy of this beautiful woman. Your mind starts flipping through every lousy tabloid tragedy ever written, by every bullshit journalist who ever lived, cutting-and-pasting bad endings onto your life. By the time you reach the crosswalk, you've convinced yourself that Fate is waiting for you in his black Trans-Am, gunning the engine, ready to do you in. Your adrenals are dumping their goodies into your system—you're mainlining pure epinephrine, much better than all the shitty coke you did in college. You grab your wife's hand, squeezing her fingers to the breaking point. You're looking left and right, to and fro, trying to see through parked cars, through corner buildings, trying to invoke X-ray vision. You fail to see the "Walk" sign, because you're staring down the guy in the black Trans-Am, who's really just some shithead from Bensonhurst, combing his hair in the rearview mirror. You feel a tug on your hand. Your wife is looking at you with worry. "Honey, it's okay to go now," she says.

You cross the street, and it begins all over again.

> *When Joseph was an old man, an old man was he*
> *He married Virgin Mary the Queen of Galilee*
> *Joseph and Mary walked through an orchard green*
> *There were berries and cherries as thick as might be seen*

And up spoke Virgin Mary so meek and so mild
Joseph gather me some cherries for I am with child
Then Joseph flew in anger, in anger flew he
"Let the father of the baby gather cherries for thee . . ."
—FROM "THE CHERRY TREE CAROL"

There is no question as to who was history's most lonely and isolated expectant father. Can you imagine? He had every right to be resentful, what with all those officious angels running about, appearing and disappearing, intruding on his dreams, issuing orders, shoving him aside. Then getting barely a mention in the Greatest Story Ever Told. Then waiting around for your pregnant wife to give birth to Jesus. What a nightmare. About all you can say for the guy is that at least he didn't have nine months of OB/GYN appointments hanging over his head.

But getting back to the larger question. Did all men feel like this when their wives were pregnant? Were these feelings of dislocation, isolation, paranoia, and brewing resentment a common theme? Maybe the story of Mary and Joseph doesn't seem like the right analogy at first glance, but when you think about it, don't men feel that their wives are being transformed? Doesn't it seem like she's on a mission from God? Doesn't it feel like some alien life form is being conjured into existence? And what exactly did you have to do with it anyway?

Since the biblical Joseph isn't around for comment, I had to turn to my friend Joseph.

"Things started to go bad about halfway through the pregnancy. It got to the point where I started wondering, 'Who is this person? What am I doing in this relationship?' I really felt that Joan had become a monster."

"A 'monster,' Joseph?" I said, trying to picture Joan with fangs or horns or green slime covering her body.

"Yes. Pregnant women are monsters of self-obsession." This from a person who would happily spend all his free time locked in a room listening to Wagner.

"I never realized the degree to which Joan could become selfish or self-centered. My recollection was always Joan saying 'my,' never 'we.' The way she talked, I had no right to the pregnancy. She simply appropriated all the emotional experience for herself, and relegated me to a subsidiary role. But on a deeper level, I had an emotional investment that I wanted and needed to express."

It's frustrating enough being a plain, ordinary male with a pregnant wife, but to be a doctor married to a pregnant doctor must be, in the immortal words of Groucho Marx, a living "pair-a-docs."

First, you have two ultra-educated, hyperanalytical, super-opinionated people going through a natural but unpredictable process and placing it under a great deal of scrutiny. (I say natural; however, they had to go through three years of an IVF program, which is in itself one of the most stressful experiences.) The husband, then, has to recuse himself from the situation—correct according to the conventions of medical ethics and procedure—but difficult and unnatural emotionally. This means that he has to distance himself from the situation while watching his partner place complete trust in yet a third ultra-educated, hyperanalytical, super-opinionated person, the OB/GYN. I can't imagine a more entangled situation than a Triangle of Doctors, especially when something so profoundly personal is at stake.

Part of the problem is also that while Joseph, intense and sensitive, was born to play Hamlet, his Ophelia has the certitude and directness of a moose, a factor that in real life, I think he would admit is good fortune for him, but in the play of his mind occasionally ruins things. I muse on these things because something seems amiss in the state of Joseph and Joan. Today we were over visiting, and I had a chance to talk to him while Julie and Joan were playing with their newborn, and out of earshot.

"We got off to a really bad start. First, she had fainting episodes. She'd always claimed to be hypoglycemic, but I was skeptical. She'd say, 'I was out shopping and I had to lie down on the sidewalk.' I made some suggestions, but I really couldn't get involved. What could I do? There were times I felt that her OB wasn't on top of things and I should do more, but it would have been unrealistic for me to hold her hand and walk her to the park and stick an IV into her every time this happened. On the other hand, I did try to show concern. I would call every morning to say, 'How are things going? How did your morning go?' But what bothers me was that by the end of the pregnancy, she felt that I had been completely uncaring during the whole time."

He stopped talking for a moment. Several rooms away, we could hear the background drone of the girls talking, occasionally punctuated with the buzzsaw of the newborn's cries. The whole situation seemed slightly dislocated, with Joseph not exactly occupying the same time and space as his wife and child.

"I felt very marginal to the experience of the pregnancy. We still went about our lives, but somehow it was very different. I felt as though Joan would be perfectly fine if she was left to herself with the fetus. The idea that she forgot, and gave no importance at all to the fact that I called every day during her fainting spells, reinforces in my mind that during that period I simply wasn't there.

"When we talked it was only about what she was experiencing. We didn't even talk politics, which is something she usually has plenty of opinions about. In the middle of one of her monologues

I could have slipped in, 'Let's starve the poor,' and she wouldn't have noticed. When I brought it to her attention, she said, 'Well it's perfectly natural, I am the center of attention.'"

Joseph paused for a moment. He was recounting his tale in an even, perfectly matter-of-fact voice, yet it was obvious that he still felt hurt and bitter about the experience. I asked him, "Do you think Joan was using the pregnancy to change the balance of power in your relationship? To take something away from you, to say this is completely mine now, and now you have to do what I want you to do."

"I have to say that when we made the decision to have the baby it was really her initiative," Joseph responded. "But this snowballed until I think she felt that the whole experience was hers alone, and that I didn't need to feel."

He went on. "When I tried to talk to her about it she would say, 'This is my role. Your role is to support me and to coach me through this, and that's what your role is, period. Our roles are distinct and mutually exclusive.'"

By this time, hearing his words resonating with my own experience, I was starting to tingle. I couldn't quite believe what I was hearing. It so directly mimicked some of my emerging fears that it seemed almost caricature-ish. I pressed on. "Why mutually exclusive?"

"She was setting emotional limits. Her attitude was, 'What I'm feeling, you can't possibly feel or understand. Even though you don't understand, you're supposed to empathize on a purely intellectual level and simply put up with me and support me.' You know, I don't think it was necessarily intentional, on her part. I think she actually felt like she was inviting me to share the pregnancy with her, but only in ways that she felt was appropriate. Basically on her own terms."

"How long did this situation go on?" I asked.

"It's still going on. But things really hit the fan at the eighteen-week ultrasound. She claimed she told me the precise day. She may very well have. It certainly didn't register and I can't recall her actually telling me. Anyway, I didn't enter it into my book. The day before she says, 'We're going to the ultrasound tomorrow,' and I said, 'Well you didn't tell me about it.' The right thing to do would have been to call my patients and say, 'I'm sorry I'm not going to be in tomorrow.' But I was so annoyed that Joan had not told me, and that at the last minute had said, 'You have got to come to this ultrasound tomorrow,' that I got my back up and said, 'I can't do this for you.' She got very angry, as you can imagine."

I decided to push him a little on this one. "That was kind of a shitty thing to do," I said.

"Okay. Looking back, I realize that I was acting out in petty ways. But you have to understand that I was disappointed in Joan and the way she was handling the pregnancy. One of the things I had always loved about her was her willingness to flout convention, her willingness to say, 'This doesn't make sense, it's just a gesture.' For example, when we got married, we had a very small wedding. Just the two of us and two witnesses. We didn't even invite our families. It was just meaningful for the two of us.

"I had expected the pregnancy to be a similar thing. Instead, every time I turned around what Joan was saying was 'I just read this book and I think it's important so you should read this.' Or, 'I just read this book and it says this is what the husband should do.' That the man's role was to wipe the woman's forehead with a washcloth, blah, blah, blah. Or, this is what a husband should be doing during the pushing period and blah, blah, blah.

"I understand that there are certain things you can do from a purely technical point of view to ease the pain or discomfort of the labor and delivery—I mean, I'm a doctor for Christ's sake!—but it seemed like throughout I was also told, 'Well, this is how you should treat me emotionally,' and throughout I really felt that we were lacking something spontaneous. I may very well have ended up doing many of those things naturally and without prodding, but it really went against my grain to be told what to do, and even worse, what to feel. We were acting out some sort of scene complete with prepackaged emotions.

"This rigidity about 'this is the woman's role, this is the man's role,' ended up making what was essentially an uneventful pregnancy very stressful. That I was expected to live up to these societal norms and expectations had the opposite effect. Instead of making me feel part of an intensely personal process, it made me feel very excluded. I bridled at being told what to do, what to think of myself, and what to feel. People have been having children for millennia and didn't rely upon some sort of owner's manual to understand what to do."

I had gotten far enough along in the pregnancy process to understand why Joseph might feel resentment, and I was even beginning to understand some of the nuances and complexities of where his resentment was coming from. But there was certainly one big thing I didn't understand: What in the world did he think the alternative was?

"That is a hard question because during the pregnancy I felt that I was constantly reacting against something. Throughout the thing I kept thinking how nice it would be if we could just be continuing our natural routine, simply continuing our lives with the only difference that Joan was pregnant. We would talk about the same things we always talked about, do the same things we always did, and get on with it. If Joan didn't have preconceived ideas of what a pregnancy should be I think we would have come to fulfill some of our own roles and been happier with the pregnancy.

"I would have loved to have felt the joy that Joan felt when she learned she was pregnant. Likewise, I wish I had understood the anxiety that Joan felt about the ultrasound, and had I not been childish I would have just canceled the appointments and gone to the ultrasound. Instead so many things got in the way."

I walked away from the visit with a feeling of poignancy. It's not every day that you open the cover of a friend's marriage to view the workings underneath. I also wondered what exactly I had learned. Some of what Joseph said seemed counterintuitive. I didn't believe that he or any man would know what to do "spontaneously." After all, despite all their talking about it, women hardly seem to know how to navigate pregnancy and birth themselves. It also seemed apparent that Joseph was angry at Joan for changing the nature of their relationship and their responsibilities. But let's face it, men often have to be dragged kicking and screaming to the next step in life after childhood. That's why all societies have manhood initiations, or similar, group-sanctioned rites of passage. Otherwise, childhood would be a party that no man would ever leave.

What I did hear and what I think was more at the heart of his complaints was an emotional disconnect that he was feeling. The pregnancy made him feel disconnected from his partner, disconnected from his coming child, and disconnected from a vision of the future. That would be enough to turn me into a raving maniac, leaving me with the only remaining logical question: Would I?

Zhoooshz . . . zhooshz . . . zhooshz . . .

I waited for Adam in the anteroom of his East Side practice, zoning out on the white noise machine that all shrinks seem to have in their offices. They probably hand them out at graduation.

Having put in more than my fair share of time in shrinks' offices over the years, I've never been able to figure out my stance on these devices. Are they meant to soothe you and lower your stress levels while you wait? Are they meant to prevent you from hearing other patients' confessions? Or are they meant to increase your stress by making you obsess about the conversations you can't hear, so that when it's your turn, you'll be ready to spill your guts?

I took him across the street to a bistro for lunch. The maître d' shoehorned us in next to a table of women in their mid-thirties. They looked up and smiled at us as we brushed past to sit down.

Adam is a friend and a successful psychotherapist with a thriving practice. In addition to couples, he has a high proportion of men in his practice, so I thought he would be a good bet to give me the skinny on what men go through during the pregnancy period, and also what effect the pregnancy experience can have on a couple's relationship. Obviously I was interested for personal reasons, but I had also begun to think that these issues would be interesting to write about. Women's magazines had started to bandy the topic about, and so I was anxious to start gathering some background information.

Adam warmed to the topic immediately. "There's a general pattern in couples or individuals with marital problems that I've noticed over the years. They start telling you the story of their lives. Sometimes people know exactly what happened and when and why. But more often it's vague, in an unconscious way, especially with men. Men come in and say, 'I no longer feel loving toward my wife, she's no longer attractive to me, or I'm infatuated with this other girl.' And then you realize, when you analyze the timeline, that the problems for many couples start during pregnancy or during the first year of parenthood."

Stories of couples breaking up shortly after the birth of a baby seem so much a part of social lore and the gossip jukebox of life that the situation seems almost archetypal. You can almost hear yourself peeling off an obligatory "I can't believe it; they seemed so happy; I feel so sorry for her and the kid" before taking another bite of a sandwich or sip of coffee. Still, hearing a therapeutic professional and a member of the "scientific community" mouth a maxim that we all feel to be intuitively true is weirdly validating. After all, we live in a time when the simplest life principle needs a documenting journal study.

"Why do you think pregnancy is ground zero for so many relationship problems?" I asked.

"Pregnancy is such a central human event. It defines the responsibilities of the genders. This makes it a powerful event for a relationship. It changes the fundamental structure and dynamic of a relationship. Men can have a variety of reactions to this. While everyone is different, I think that certain reactions can be characterized as universal. For example, a feeling of abandonment."

I told Adam some of the details of Joseph's experience with Joan. "Do you think Joseph was going through this?"

"When two becomes three, there's often trouble. We all know that one of the fundamental ideas of psychoanalysis is that three is when conflict starts, the whole Oedipal thing. This dynamic starts in pregnancy, when the mother gets very attached to the fetus, leaving the man feeling abandoned and excluded."

What about Joseph's complaint that Joan took all the emotional content of the pregnancy for herself?

"Pregnancy is all about the power of women, and this raises many issues for men. In your friend's case I think this comes through in a couple of ways. All men have a feminine side . . ."

"You mean like Dennis Rodman or Marv Albert?" I blurted out. We both took a moment to share a chuckle.

"My practice is full of men with sexual dysfunctions, and I can tell you that it's the most hypermasculine of men who often have the strongest need to be feminine. But anyway, your friend's need to have some emotional stake in the pregnancy, as he puts it, perhaps represents his desire to be the 'mother,' to take part in the female narrative. This unfortunately places him in direct competition with his partner, who obviously has her own ideas and expectations about what he should be doing. Which leads to a larger point: Men are prevented from exploring the fullness of their emotional existence because of the expectations of society, and ironically because of the expectations of women."

What about Joseph's complaint that he resented not only Joan's expectations, but also society's expectations of what the father's role should be like?

"Men's roles as 'men' aren't the only thing restricted by social conventions; men are also still hemmed in by society's expectation's of what fatherhood is. This is something that feminists don't really adequately understand: A 'man's role' is also a burden to men. Men suffer as much as women do from this so-called male superiority and sexual discrimination. Men, in my practice and in general, feel that they are not part of the game when it comes to children. Men go to work, they do the providing thing, and then they feel excluded. Women raise the children, they don't consult men about what to do, they don't give men a say."

And so what happens? Men act out by not showing up to ultrasounds?

"Worse, much worse. Whereas women are much more introspective, much more relationship-, communication-, and process-oriented, men act out and have 'symptoms.' During pregnancy or the first year of the baby's life, many men have affairs, some abuse drugs, others abandon their wives. I don't know what the statistics are, but I also think that the incidence of domestic violence might increase."

"Yikes!" I thought. "This is sounding grim." I was beginning to have visions of myself being dragged away by the police, foaming at the mouth, with needles dangling from my arm, clutching a bottle of single malt to my chest. I also couldn't help but notice that the women at the adjoining table were also taking great interest in our little talk. It was subtle, but I could sense them "leaning in" to our conversation. Occasionally I would even catch a quick glance or see a tiny smile or smirk.

I also remembered that Adam's wife, Mimi, was a psychotherapist, too. Now if there's anything I could imagine more difficult than two doctors going through a pregnancy, it's two therapists. I had to ask him.

"Adam, what was your pregnancy experience like?"

The question made him instantly nervous. I could tell by the way he started dipping his finger in his salad dressing and drawing designs on my tape recorder.

"Mimi and I were together for five years before she became pregnant. We had a very intense relationship and we devoted a lot of time to each other. Maybe some people would be better off not knowing each other as well or as long. If people get married after six months and have a child two months later, they never have this experience to lose. They have other stuff to deal with.

"Anyway, I had a really hard time during Mimi's pregnancy. I had a lot of feelings, which took me years to understand. In fact, we're still dealing with it. I felt that she was abandoning me for this other person, and it made me very, very angry."

How angry?

"I was very critical of her. A lot of things she did bothered me. I hated the way she looked. Instead of being supportive, I told her all of these things. It was bad because I really didn't take care of her emotionally. I was having my own rageful pregnancy."

"Why did you just call it your 'own rageful pregnancy'?"

"This stuff was coming out of nowhere. I was harboring these feelings of anger and resentment and they were building up. These thoughts would come up. They wouldn't seem to be mine, but they would be irrepressible. People have obsessive thoughts that emerge, fantasies. I think this was my equivalent of it. I felt that this was something that was hostile toward me, so I became hostile. I wasn't really very conscious of it. I didn't want to show it, but I did. I use this term because it felt like I was pregnant with this anger."

"So, what were some of your fantasies?"

"I wanted to punch pregnant woman in the stomach," he said, punching the air for emphasis.

That did it. The table of women next to us were craning their necks, like overstimulated swans, hanging on our every word. Over the course of the next hour as Adam and I continued our talk, they were practically sitting in our laps. We were better than Oprah.

> In the misfortune of our best friends we often find something not displeasing.
> —François, Duc de La Rochefoucauld (1613–1680)

"Hi, Gordon? It's Gary."

"Hey, what's up? How's Louise?"

"Louise is in labor. We're at the hospital. I need a favor."

"Sure, anything. Name it."

If there is anything more pleasurable than doing a friend in need a favor, it's the pleasure that one feels that the friend is in a position of needing you in the first place. I'm thinking of the German word *Schadenfreude*—my all-time favorite expression—which basically means "feeling pleasure at the misfortune of others." *Schadenfreude*—and its twin sister "jealousy of another's good fortune"—are my favorites because, despite what we would like to believe about ourselves, they are the most reliable of human reactions. Almost instinctual. (Then there's also the need to say, "I told you so.")

My evil doppelgänger twin entertained these thoughts while the real me sat across from my best friend, Gary, in New York Hospital's commissary trying my best to be comforting and supportive. Gary called me earlier to ask me to come to the hospital and pick up their car and return it to their house, as he expected they would be a while.

Outside, New York Hospital is beautiful—with attitude. When you approach the main entrance, you see a huge gothic arch, framed by brushed aluminum and cast bas-relief that resemble gorgeous hood ornaments. These are shining statements of confidence, and it's comforting to feel that some part of your society is so sure of itself that they would actually stick little logos on something as dodgy and terminal as a hospital.

We went up to Labor and Delivery. Louise was resting on her back on a gurney, her knees cocked up in the air, slightly akimbo, her feet resting on stirrups. Loosely straddling the huge globe of her waist, a wide belt with a huge buckle: the electronic monitoring. Stacked over her head were telemetry monitors measuring her vital signs and the vital signs of the fetus. Her eyes were squeezed shut—part of an overall grimace that held her face hostage—and in the cold light of the overhead fluorescent tubes, her skin was gray.

There's nothing like being reduced to being a barnyard animal at your own nativity. Gary ushered me into a corner and we both tried to make ourselves the size of mice, as the occasional intern or resident would trickle into the room to do something relatively useless. As they entered the room they looked at us with irritation, as if somehow being the husband of the delivering woman didn't quite justify Gary's existence. There is a golden rule that should be applied to medical supernumeraries: Attitude is usually in inverse proportion to actual experience. If you have spent as much time in hospitals consulting or shooting documentaries as I have, you know that many of the people hovering officiously around bedside have less experience tending to sick people than, say, flight attendants. It's enough to make you want to run screaming from them as they come at you with something as simple as a thermometer.

Which only served to counterpoint the situation. In normal life, meaning his job, Gary is a star. He is on the fast track at one of the largest media conglomerates in the world. He elevates effectiveness to brilliance. His temperament, for which he is much prized by his bosses and feared by his competitors and subordinates, is an iceberg: The cool inscrutability of his surface is more than matched by the implacable, ship-killing gravity of the part you can't see. Here is a person who can fire fifty people in an afternoon, withstand the temper tantrum of a group president, seal a $100 million deal, and make it home to cook his wife dinner. And yet in this situation, I could tell, he felt uncomfortable and powerless.

We did the only thing we could do; we left to get a tuna fish sandwich.

"It's all bullshit. This Lamaze stuff, it's just total bullshit," Gary said, mayonnaise dribbling onto his chin.

"It didn't work?" I said, between bites, trying my best to sound genuinely incredulous and sympathetic, when I really hadn't the faintest idea what Lamaze is.

"Three sessions of hee-hee-hee breathing, and when the moment comes to apply it, your wife arches her back at the first real contraction, looks at you with dark satanic eyes, and you know instantly it's useless and stupid. What are you supposed to say after that? More ice chips, dear?"

"It didn't work at all? Not even a little?"

"Nada. And OBs certainly don't give a shit about it. They're like: If you're in pain, take an epidural. And if we don't get dilation of the cervix, we do a C-section. They're real ho-hum about it."

"How long have you been here?"

"Oh, about eighteen hours."

Eighteen hours. My mind slowly circled the concept, as if an alien ship had just landed in front of me. Eighteen hours in a state of anxiety and pain. In a world of Access on-demand to off-the-shelf Zen, it seemed an unthinkable amount of time to spend inconvenienced. They must be doing something wrong, I thought.

It was especially ironic if you knew what Gary and Louise went through to get here; that their slow-moving labor and delivery experience was preceded by one of the most high-tech pregnancies on record. Gary and Louise's parenting plans were complicated by the fact that Gary is missing a vital piece of equipment, his vas deferens, the tiny duct that connects the epididymis, the part of the testicle that makes sperm, with the ejaculatory duct. In other words, Gary shoots blanks—something he would have loved to have known during his dating years.

"If we had discovered this even a year before, there would have been no recourse but to adopt or to go to a sperm bank," Gary said, describing how proud of himself the fertility specialist had seemed while relating this information. Because of their timing, Gary and Louise had the opportunity to take part in one of the first attempts at epididymal marsupialization. What this involved was doctors performing surgery to create a little sac inside his scrotum near the epididymal structure, called a Moni window. The idea was that sperm cells created by the epididymis would slowly pool and collect in this sac. I used to tease Gary by telling him that the surgery put him in the same class as possums, kangaroos, wombats, and Tasmanian devils.

Then came the good part. At two- to three-week intervals in procedures of two to three hours in duration, an elite cadre of reproductive specialists and surgeons, guided by ultrasound imaging, would extract the sperm using their tool of choice—a four-inch needle—without anesthesia. As Gary loved to explain with calculated insouciance, the doctors offered him a local, but he turned it down. The extra liquid volume created by the addition of anesthesia would complicate finding the Moni window. So he did without.

Now, if this sounds like a procedure performed with the precision of modern science, it wasn't. It was more like an ice fishing expedition conducted by blind Inuits, gathered around a hole cut in Gary's scrotum, stabbing with their harpoons. Six times they did this without success. With each failure, ever more important layers of reproductive righteousness were added, until the seventh procedure featured the chairman of the department and his archangels sweating over Gary's swollen testicles.

Oh, and the pain. Here virility inverted itself. Gary couldn't have children the normal way, but what he had to go through to have them artificially required far more machismo than any other males I can think of, including Ultimate Fighters, Hell's Angels, and Navy Seals. "The third time I had it done," he said, "I was in so much pain that I couldn't leave the doctor's office. I had to sit there for two hours on a couch, practicing my deep breathing so I wouldn't throw up, before I could get myself into a cab."

I watched as Gary continued methodically eviscerating his soggy sandwich. It felt weird, the two of us "men" sitting in a nasty little cafeteria, gnawing on bad tuna, while Louise was going through incredible pain four floors above. I felt genuine compassion for her and for Gary, but what also amazed me was my own detachment. A thirty-second AT&T commercial can leave one in tears, but the travails of a best friend, they are to be studied with the detachment worthy of frog dissection. What can it say about human nature?

Maybe it says that friendship often has as much to do with competition as it has to do with love. As a person, Gary is like a brother to me, but as social beings we compete ferociously. I have always seemed to be the one to take more risks. I am outwardly more flamboyant. He is cool and reserved. I chose an unconventional "career path." He became a corporate tool. But the reality may be somewhat different. He got married first. I followed, three weeks later. He moved to Park Slope first. A year later, I followed. He and Louise decided to have children. Six months later, Julie was pregnant.

Of course, as you get older the competition intensifies, especially as everyone "couples up." People begin to notice differences in lifestyles, salaries, houses, cars, vacations: the choices you have, or don't have. This also extends to an acquired knowledge base, a life "expertise," how well one is perceived at making strategic decisions. Couples are forever looking at each other and clucking, "How do they get by? How do they survive?"

There is one place that Gary did go that I didn't. Three years ago he had an affair that almost ended his marriage. It happened after the first time he and Louise had tried to get pregnant (this was before Gary found out about his condition). After trying for a year without success, they took a little break from baby making, chalking up the lack of results to Louise's history of ovarian cysts and scarring from surgery. During this hiatus, Gary started seeing a younger woman, a colleague at work. Eventually he confessed to Louise. It got very, very messy.

He came to live with us for several months. I sat through many drunken conversations in which Gary tried to decide whether to end his marriage or go back to Louise. I remember once arguing with him, trying to get him to see the classic situation he had created, a situation that begged for armchair Sunday afternoon Freudianism and Monday night sociobiology. "Here's scenario number one," I said. "You want kids. You're having trouble having kids with Louise. At the same time, you say you don't really respect your spouse as much as you wish you did because of her personality and her job. So you choose a younger, more vibrant, and metaphorically fertile women; it's a natural thing. Scenario number two, you're freaked out by the baby-making process. You're ambivalent about taking this next step with Louise, because you have ambivalent feelings about her. So you act out by having an affair."

Of course he denied everything. He denied that any of it had anything to do with what was going on in his life at the time, leaving him with explanations like pure, blind lust and plain stupidity. Eventually he went back to Louise. His reasons?

"I had basically turned on the fantasy mill, big-time. When I finally woke up I realized that the very qualities that I really wanted weren't present in Terri. A more youthful person wasn't going to translate into the kind of commitment, security, and strong relationship that I really wanted."

Case closed.

Of course there was one little problem: Louise's anger. There was no doubt in my mind that she understood the nature and symbolism of Gary's betrayal. Yet, to our amazement—meaning Julie, me, and mutual friends—several months after reconciling, they were trying again to get pregnant. Few of us thought it was a good idea; it was just too soon. And when I found out that they needed IVF, I thought that they would never make it. If IVF stressed healthy relationships to the limit, what would it do to their wounded one?

I remember Gary telling me that he knew what the risks were, that "we realized the program could be our worst nightmare, that it could be like walking into a meat grinder. Instead, it brought us together."

Perhaps making a baby in this way provided a practical means to reknit the seemingly infinite tendrils of emotion and history that flowed openly into the atmosphere when their marriage knot burst. It also gave them the kind of intimacy that only develops around dangerous work. Two shots a day in the ass of Mediprin and Perganol for a total of four weeks. For Gary: It meant he had to really pay attention to Louise. As for Louise: When someone is jabbing a three-inch needle into your butt, no matter what he's done, you have to find a way to trust.

In the end, the Gary's level of physical participation in the pregnancy became symbolic in a way that most men don't get to experience. When you think about it, the pain he went through to "deliver" his sperm so that they could have kids at all foreshadowed her own pregnancy. As Gary liked to say, he "had his pregnancy first," and I think it was this "birth experience" that sealed the bond. I can remember how Louise, with considerable satisfaction, related Gary's reaction after the seventh Moni window extraction attempt. Louise, who had accompanied Gary to the procedure, broke the news that the doctors had finally hit pay dirt. "I told him, 'Sweetie, they got 60 million sperm!' Gary lost control and cried."

It was time to go back to Louise on the fourth floor. I couldn't stay much longer. Julie and I had a long-standing commitment to go to Washington and visit friends for the weekend. Part of me was sorry that I couldn't stay and keep Gary company; part of me was quite happy to go. I walked him back to the labor room where Louise was sleeping fitfully with the help of an epidural. Standing there quietly for a moment with Gary, I had a small epiphany. Another reason occurred to me for this odd sense of detachment I had felt during my visit: We study the lives of our friends to measure the risk in our own. Looking down at her, the future looked complicated.

I gave Gary a hug and kissed him on the cheek. Then I went on my way.

Taking a pee in a sterile white bathroom, I see a row of Dixie cups containing urine samples lining the counter above the sink. It's like being stuck in the yellow section of a large Crayola box: The colors range from "Straw" to "Burnt Sienna." Each one has been labeled with a big blue Sharpie. I search out my wife's sample. "Pumpkin Chiffon." Mental note: "Needs to drink more water."

Going to your wife's OB/GYN appointment has become a big rite of passage for men. I know this because, while men don't talk about it explicitly, it is always mentioned in conversations about pregnancy, like wearing a verbal tag showing that the speaker is a with-it husband. Another indicator of how important this rite has become: A lot of men miss the first appointment. I know I did. What can I say? Denial must work in mysterious ways. Luckily, Julie didn't make too much of it.

But here I am at the second appointment, present and accounted for. The truth is, I was really looking forward to it. Unlike many people, I have a great love of bodily functions of all sorts. I also have a healthy interest in female genitals that I can trace back to a day when all the girls in the sixth grade were trotted off to watch films about menstrual flow and what-not, while us boys had to be satisfied with word-of-mouth information about our peckers. Finally, I was looking forward to visiting the sanctum sanctorum, the holy of holies of femaledom, where I could watch the ministrations of that select priestess cult, the doctors of gynecology. (Male GYNs are a dying breed, for obvious reasons.)

If men aren't quite ready to venture into women's most sacred enclave, there are signs that women aren't that comfortable with them being there. First of all, there is the overabundance of car magazines in the waiting room. I felt as if I had returned to my childhood. Here were *Road & Track*, *Car & Driver*, *Automobile*—even *Petersen's 4X4*. But why? Had I stumbled onto a GYN practice entirely made up of a cult of woman car enthusiasts? Or was this evidence of a universal female obsession that remained a secret from me and all the other men on the planet? If only I had known when I was dating. Even now, I could envision Julie and I growing old talking about that seminal moment in my childhood: the introduction, in 1969, of the Pontiac Superbird.

Alas no. The truth is far less intriguing. This is merely what the all-female office staff think that men like and need, to get them through the experience of the visit. Must the genders infantilize each other to get along? Why not make it real simple? Just hand me some good pornography and a flashlight.

The second sign was Dr. Spyros's mild discomfort when I tagged along to the exam room. I take nothing away from her;

after all she was the person who answered the page at 4 A.M. on Easter morning with perfect equanimity. But I could tell from her reaction that most men, when they say they'll go with their wives to the appointment, mean that they'll sit in the waiting room while the doctor pops the hood.

I parked myself in an out-of-the-way corner of the exam room. Julie mounted the exam table with all the poise of an astronaut ascending the gantry to the Apollo capsule. Dr. Spyros stripped on a pair of latex gloves and inserted a speculum to hold open Julie's vagina. Next she inserted a long tubular scope with a light on the end and spent a few minutes viewing the insides through an eyepiece. For a moment I fantasized that Spyros was some sort of astronomer, a Galileo charting a newly discovered inner universe—a reverie that came to a crashing halt when she then proceeded to stick one hand deep into Julie's vagina to feel her cervix. I flinched and grimaced. This was more like unstopping a plugged sink drain. It did not look at all pleasant, but Julie seemed unconcerned.

After a few comments to Julie about the state of her insides, Spyros pulled out a transducer connected to an ultrasound machine. She turned to me and smiled, motioning me closer. She glopped a huge dollop of K-Y Jelly onto the transducer and skated the head of the instrument over Julie's abdomen. Suddenly the room filled with sound: a loud, roaring *shoo . . . shoo . . . shoo.* We all looked expectantly at the machine's screen, which flickered several times and then flared into an image.

Here was my inner universe. And there, off the shoulder of a necklace of stars slung like pearly vertebrae, appeared a ship with a beating smudge of a heart as its beacon. At the controls, our tiny nameless pilot, racing toward us at speeds beyond my comprehension.

MONTH FOUR

OF SEA HORSES
AND THE COUVADE

Okay, so now it's official. Julie and I are sitting in Monica and PJ's kitchen. It's a cold midwinter day. Out of their bay window, I can see their garden. While Monica boils water for tea and does girl talk with Julie, I'm overtaken by involuntary reverie. I remember sitting out there surrounded by the lushness of last summer, enjoying a glass of wine at brunch, immersed in conversation and a cloud bank of rose scent. Now, their garden is a symbol of loss, as if someone pulled a snowy pool cover over my life. The brilliant conversation table is a white shapeless lump, the rose bushes reduced to a few desultory stalks. All seems formless and incomprehensible. I now understand why cordless bungee jumping is the Scandinavian national sport. I cheer myself up momentarily by looking over at Julie and imagining her as a large, dormant, tulip bulb. It's not difficult, at this point. The teakettle whistles. Monica brews Earl Grey and my mind goes back to brewing its own dark and mysterious liquor.

What's official is my resentment. Up until this point, I've kept to vague feelings of displacement and discontent. Now, Monica has given me an article describing something called the Empathy Belly Pregnancy Simulator. It's a few pages torn out of a parenting magazine—an idea that makes my eyes glaze over, every month a new toddler centerfold—showing a male talk show host wearing a prosthesis in the shape of a huge belly and breasts. The net effect is a sort of Botero Frankenstein, if you can imagine. The device weighs thirty-three pounds, is filled with lead shot and water, and "allows the wearer to experience up to 20 different symptoms of pregnancy, including backaches, bladder pressure, increased body temperature, and 'fetal kicks,' delivered when an internal lead weight bounces against the body."

"I created the Empathy Belly to increase men's understanding of pregnancy," says the inventor. A secondary motive, she adds, "was to dismiss male misconceptions that pregnancy is not all that hard."

Somehow I feel deflated. I've been trying very hard to feel excited about the pregnancy—desperately been trying to go beyond merely the pat-on-the-back stage and actually find some meaning in all this beyond metaphors for the efficacy of saturation bombing. What really bothers me is that I'm getting this reaction of seeming ridicule from women whom I consider my "buddies." Monica is someone I relate to and confide in irrespective of gender. I know she means well, but something about the picture of this guy wearing this device is ultimately and immediately humiliating. The other day, Maggie from Dublin did the same thing to me. When I mentioned some of the feelings I've had about the pregnancy, she laughed loudly, made some choking noises, and had to put down the phone.

So much for the vaunted empathy of women. I should have known better than to have trusted the opposite sex with my feelings.

What does it mean? Why does the picture of the talk show host wearing the Empathy Belly Pregnancy Simulator irritate me so much? I'm not sure I totally understand the feelings fully, but let me give it a try. The picture says this to me: "If you are a man you have no understanding of what women go through, and if you did, you would have no appreciation; if you want to gain some under-standing of pregnancy you first have to understand and appreciate how much we suffer." In one sense, I don't have a problem with any of this. I tend to be ignorant of what women go through, could probably use a lesson in gender humility, and need to dedicate more time to thinking about my partner's feelings. In other words, I accept that as a man I need to be beaten regularly with a big stick. Joking aside, I can comprehend the idea that the profound body changes a woman goes through are central to the experience and meaning of pregnancy—for women.

Increasing men's understanding of pregnancy may be another story. The central issue here is: What meaning can a man draw from the pregnancy period which will prepare him to be a caring and helpful partner and a good father? The answer to that ques-tion, my friends, is not going to be found in what is happening to the woman's body.

The problem continues. Women today want men to be com-pletely with-it fathers to the point where we're expected to wade arm-in-arm through the hip-deep guano of nurseries, test boil-ing hot formula on the skins of our forearms, puzzle together over the abomination of preschool applications. Yet after 1.6 million years of being nowhere near the child-raising scene, we males are expected to read a few books, attend a few classes, and get right with it. I'm afraid I need a little more preparation before I can say, "Gymboree, here I come!"

The fact that women want men to be full partners in the

child-raising process, and yet don't understand that a man might be searching for meaning for himself during the pregnancy process, is in itself meaningful. Surely the meaningfulness of pregnancy doesn't come down to wearing thirty-three pounds of lead shot on your chest, does it? Saying so would only prove that women today are still imprisoned by the same view of society that men have engendered. If men are slackards in inventing intelligent strategies that lead to fuller and more satisfying coop-eration between the sexes, so are women.

Do men really think that pregnancy isn't that hard? One of the things really setting me off, I am realizing, is how much physical risk pregnancy entails. Nature chose wrongly as far as I'm con-cerned. Physical risk, pain, and other humiliations of the body are the daily coin of every man's upbringing. He understands and is on intimately familiar terms with it from the time he watches his best buddy catch a Little League baseball in the teeth. So, far from dis-missing pregnancy as "not all that hard," I actually can't compre-hend how Julie is going to get through this experience with her basic training as a girl. I mean, I didn't notice any Childbirth Bar-bies being clutched by little girls on the bus, did you?

It's confused, and irrational, but it's true—some twisted part of me really thinks I can do a better job of being pregnant.

The other day I was walking Julie down the street, holding on to her hand, when I had this strange vision. I was doing my usual guard dog thing, calculating the vectors of large moving objects and using my X-ray vision to peer through parked cars and buildings when a thought occurred to me with all the subtlety of the Annunciation. What if a terrible accident occurred at the next corner? What if a gang of violent hoods had broken into the bank we were just in, and sprayed the lobby with bullets? What if Julie was critically wounded? What if I had to choose between

Julie's life and the life of the baby? Logic tells me that I should choose Julie's life. She is young enough; we could make other children together. But, a few steps later, a strange impulse within me opts for the child, and for a block or two, I fantasize about raising the child myself.

How's that for empathy belly?

I've never actually held a conference call via speakerphone from the comfort of my own kitchen, but if you've already got the technology in place, why not? I have newfound respect for that beige piece of crap I've been abusing all these years. Who knew it had a speakerphone?

In a scene out of bad performance art, Julie and I have the phone in the middle of the kitchen table and we're taking turns shouting at it. Our other kitchen appliances are looking on with great interest. The phone is talking back to us with the voice of a genetics counselor from a testing lab recommended by our OB.

They're going to analyze the results of the amniocentesis we've scheduled later on in the month.

Sometimes convenience doesn't pay off. Something tells me we should have gone for a face-to-face like Dr. Spyros had recommended and not opted for the telephone interview. This is not exactly the touchy-feely experience that I had envisioned—the one where the counselor soothingly tells us that there is nothing to worry about and that our child is not going to be born with something that qualifies us for a television movie of the week. Also, the genetics counselor doesn't seem to understand her role vis-à-vis my emotional state, or maybe it's just the Tin Man disembodiment that the speakerphone is creating.

Is it just me or is anyone else struck by the perversity of information? Did people in times before us actually worry this much about what could possibly happen? We live in a genetics-mad world. The airwaves are obese with "special reports" on diseases and conditions with possible genetic linkages. Every couple of months or so, the *New York Times* Science section reports on the Human Genome Project with the breathlessness usually saved for Tom Cruise.

What makes it particularly perverse is that these ideas have an impact on our lives, but we have no control over them. Once we gave ourselves a degree of personal control and dignity by dealing with that which we could not control through myths, religions, and philosophy. Now science is the sole storyteller. Being a good rationalist, I have no problem with science being the primary source of knowledge, except for the fact that science, since it is a series of arguments and counterarguments, is ultimately a lousy storyteller. The narrative is constantly being interrupted for 180-degree revisions: All humans evolved from the same population; humans evolved from several populations. Dietary fat leads to coronary artery disease; dietary fat is not as bad as we thought. The effect is Kafka-esque, with most of us parked in the Great Waiting Room, sipping cappuccino, anticipating the latest press release from the authorities.

Of course, the speakerphone knows that this centrifuge of doubt and neurosis whirs at the center of each individual, and so compensates accordingly.

"I want to start off by asking you to remember that you have a 97 percent chance of having a normal child. That is an overwhelming number for success. That leaves a 3 percent chance of deviation, which is a very small number. Because of Julie's family background, we'll test for Tay-Sachs and Gaucher's disease. Also, at your request we're doing a test for cystic fibrosis. Basically, with the amnio, we'll be looking at all forty-six chromosomes to see if there are any additions or deletions. We'll do an alpha-fetoprotein to make sure there are no open neural tube defects. Again, the procedure is very safe. Some women experience vaginal cramping for a couple of hours after the procedure. Less than half a percent of all women who undergo this procedure experience complications that lead to miscarriage. A very small number."

At this point I was beginning to think we had Glinda, the Good Bookmaker of the North, on our hands.

My little mind was racing, desperately trying to remember eleventh grade biology with Mrs. Reilly. What I remember most about this section of the curriculum—believe me, I'm amazed that I remember anything at all—is a bunch of kids crowded around a book possibly called *Human Reproduction and Genetics*. Of course what we were all interested in was the chapter on birth defects and genetic abnormalities. From these pages stared out at us a parade of unfortunates who, through no responsibility of their own, had been left to the mercy of an inept creator or random mutation, depending on your perspective, and who were posed and displayed in a quaintly nineteenth-century style that I will describe as photographic formaldehyde. What is ironic, thinking back from my present vantage point, is how many in that crowd of "normal" children went on to suffer from some defect in judgment, character, and personality, resulting in social costs such as divorce, depression, welfare, and jail time, and yet we were almost uniformly united by our morphological disgust and amusement and our choruses of "Ooh, gross!"

"Do you have any questions for me?" squawked the speakerphone.

"Yes," I said. "Why can't we screen for all possible genetic problems?"

"Well," replied the speakerphone, "in order to do that, we

would run out of amniotic fluid and money. There is no such thing as a 'gene screen' at the moment. The forty-six chromosomes we'll be examining contain over 100,000 genes, and at the moment there are nearly 4,000 possible genetic abnormalities and diseases that we know about. So the important point of what we're doing today is to get a complete family history so that we can narrow down the possibilities. Mr. Churchwell, were you able to find out if your younger brother was a case of trisomy-21 or translocation?"

Ah, now it comes back to me. One of the things that bothered me about the scene from Mrs. Reilly's class. One of the faces staring out at me is a likeness of my own brother, John.

DOWN'S SYNDROME, TRISOMY-21, or (formerly) MONGOLISM, congenital disorder caused by an extra chromosome on the chromosome twenty-one pair, thus giving the person a total of forty-seven chromosomes rather than the normal forty-six. Persons born with Down's syndrome are characterized by several of the following: broad, flat face; short neck; up-slanted eyes, sometimes with an inner epicanthal fold; low-set ears; small nose and enlarged tongue and lips; sloping underchin; poor muscle tone; mental retardation; heart or kidney malformations or both; and abnormal dermal ridge patterns on fingers, palms, and soles. The mental retardation seen in persons with Down's syndrome is usually moderate, though in some it may be mild or severe.

When people say the amnio represents a complicated issue for them, I laugh.

It's amazing how quickly, when confronted with the limitations of knowledge, we revert "scientific" problems to metaphysical ones. Not being able to control what happens in the creation process defaults to all kinds of squishy questions such as "How good a person am I?" as if somehow raking through the moral entrails of your life will yield some augury to your chances of breeding a "perfectly healthy" or "normal" child versus a "damaged" one. Everyone then succumbs to a Catholic parody of the Mendelian process where "Done Good" genes yield "normal," while "Done Bad" genes could yield imperfection. Then other, more protective and slightly less suspect rationalizations will creep in, such as "Won't raising handicapped people make us a better, less selfish, and more moral people, and by extension, society? Aren't mentally retarded people really saints in disguise?"

I do not feel that my brother is a gift from God, nor do I have any other concept for him that can be neatly tied with a bow. He is my brother. He is incredibly irritating at times, stubborn, likes to have his own way, watches way too much television, eats too much, can't control many of his impulses, interrupts in the middle of conversations, doesn't always bathe or shave, and so on. Which is to say he is remarkably like me, except that he is also fastidiously responsible, has been steadily employed since leaving high school, saves money and is otherwise fiscally conservative, and is generally tolerant of and welcoming to people that he meets in the course of his daily life. But to say that he is simply my brother is also to be disingenuous.

I have seen the enormous resources that had to go into my brother's life. In 1962, amniocentesis was nonexistent. I do not know how my parents felt when they realized John had what was known then as mongolism, but in a time when Down's children were routinely institutionalized, my parents chose a much more difficult path. No one else believed he would ever amount to anything, so my parents literally had to pioneer programs at the local school district, cajoling and threatening the powers-that-be in order to get them to provide my brother with speech therapy, and invent special education programs for the disabled. All without the help of support groups.

What did we learn as a family? What did we gain? Learning and gaining may be two different things. My brother required and will always require more than his share of attention. My parents did not spend as much time on their relationship as they should have and have drifted apart. The youngest, my little sister, who followed John, became painfully shy and withdrawn. As for myself, I have always felt deprived of the feeling that my siblings are my companions.

So be it. All I know is that I just crave a little normalcy, whatever that is.

Speakerphone, do all people worry the way I do about what will happen if they give birth to a defective child?

"Yes all people worry, but New Yorkers worry more. You all seem to worry twice as much as the rest of the country. I mean it's not the same in Peoria."

Yeah, probably not. It would be interesting to know what the real figures are like.

"I already know. It's not the same in Peoria. There are studies. I've read them and I've been there."

How did we men get our reputation for ineptness?

You don't have to look much further than television. I'm doing some research at today's version of the Great Library of Alexandria, the Museum of Television and Radio. Inside the heavily carpeted precincts of the museum's library, one is greeted and ushered to a computer terminal by a staff of implausibly fresh-faced *90210* docents who are friendly and pleasant, but strike me as people who think that Sancho Panza is the Dalai Llama's press representative.

Once I am seated at a terminal, the feeling of power is inescapable. The secrets of American life amortized over nearly a half-century of exploration and storytelling, hundreds of thousands of episodes, billions of dollars of expenditure, the minds of countless scriptwriters, producers, and directors. Everything cross-referenced and cross-correlated through a multitude of genres, formats, and sensibilities. Surely, this is one of history's better engines for thought and investigation. Imagine the possibilities! I am almost tempted to type in "W-H-E-N W-I-L-L T-H-E K-N-I-C-K-S W-I-N T-H-E N-B-A C-H-A-M-P-I-O-N-S-H-I-P?" but decide to stick with my plan, and punch in "P-R-E-G-N-A-N-C-Y" instead.

The computer chews on this query for an interminable five minutes or so, and then returns a list of hundreds of television programs. As I laboriously start reading the program synopses, what's immediately apparent is how central reproduction is to the dramatic and comedic richness of American life. Pregnancy is obviously a great plot device because reproduction leads to so many complications. Get a woman pregnant, stick her into heaps of trouble, and you've got an instant show.

After about an hour of wading, I make my selections and proceed to the viewing room, a bizarre space filled with television monitors and VCRs. Here, in a public phosphor bath, people gather to revisit the favorite television moments of their life. In Booth #3, a septuagenarian with a Boca leather tan laughs hearty lungfuls at Sid Caesar's *Show of Shows*. Booth #14, a fortyish woman in a power suit has a date with Greg of *The Brady Bunch*. Over in Booth #38, a Gen-X semiotician reviews the brief and ample Jenny McCarthy *oeuvre*. I punch a code number into the VCR. A big black-and-white valentine fills the screen.

The best of the lot is *I Love Lucy*. Lucy, very pregnant,

announces that the doctor has said the baby could arrive at any moment. Ricky freaks out. Lucy then explains that "at any moment" could be several days. Ricky sits and stares at Lucy in anticipation, driving her crazy. Fred and Ethel arrive. Fred, Ethel, and Ricky calmly rehearse for the hospital trip. When Lucy announces that she is having contractions, the three panic. Next scene. Lucy walks into hospital admitting. Ricky follows slumped in a wheelchair. He is almost completely incapacitated.

Things get really weird. Ricky after pacing for a while in the waiting room, *goes to his club*—now we know we're in the fifties—and gets into hideous-looking voodoo makeup and outfit to do his act. In the middle of the number he gets a message that the baby has arrived. He returns to the hospital looking like a savage in his voodoo costume. Fred bumps into him and faints. The police come and grab Ricky. Finally everything gets straightened out. A frightened nurse appears to tell Ricky: "They're bringing your baby boy to the window." Ricky goes to the nursery window, looks upon his newborn child, and faints. Babalu!

The hit parade of ineptitude continues. In a *Flintstones* episode Fred and pregnant Wilma are in bed when Fred, with his usual bravado, says: "I just want you to know I'm ready! Can I get you some pickles?" Wilma asks for a glass of water and sets Fred off.

FRED: Water? You don't know nothing about having a baby.

WILMA: Oh, Fred, will you relax.

FRED: Oh, sure, sure. All you have to do is tell me you're ready and your job's done.

WILMA: And what do you have to do?

FRED: Are you kidding? I have to call the doctor, come and get your suitcase, drive to the hospital—you're hardly involved in this thing at all.

WILMA: I had no idea what you fathers go through. This could take several days, you'll be a nervous wreck.

FRED (protesting): Me nervous? Don't worry, I'm one father who's going to remain calm. (He then proceeds to literally wear a groove in the floor.) This waiting, waiting, waiting is tough!

The *Dick Van Dyke Show* opens with Rob and pregnant Laura Petrie in bed. Laura turns to say something to an obviously very skittish Rob. Rob bounds out of bed. He's got his business suit on. Rob has been sleeping in his suit in order to be ready to take Laura to the hospital.

An almost unwatchable *Odd Couple* episode has Felix escorting his obviously much younger and pregnant wife to the hospital, where he manages to irritate the hospital staff to the point where they're almost literally ready to murder him.

Strangest is an early black-and-white *Cosby Special* with a skit where Bill Cosby and Herb Edelman play two pregnant men! The scene opens with a pregnant Edelman waiting in a labor room. An orderly wheels in Cosby. There they lay in adjacent beds with huge bulbous bellies. Both of them are smoking cigars.

EDELMAN: Is this your first? If you knew what you're going to go through you wouldn't be smiling. (Laugh.) "When the pain starts. . . . How often do they come?
(Cosby starts moaning.)
EDELMAN: Take it easy, there's really nothing to worry about. Some guys make a big deal out of it. But there's really nothing to it.
COSBY: You know my wife wanted to stay and watch me.
EDELMAN: So did mine, but I wouldn't let her. She hasn't looked at me in three months, why should I let her look at me now. How long did you stay on the job?

COSBY (puffing on his cigar): I stayed as long as I could and then I found it hard to hide the "showing" from my boss. Should I call the doctor or the nurse?

EDELMAN: There is nothing to worry about. (Then he starts arching his back and yelling in pain.) Nurse! Nurse! Estelle, why did you do this to me?

NURSE (black male): Did somebody call for a nurse? Oh really, Mr. "False Alarm" Edelman. Do you know how many men are having babies today? Will you just relax? By the way, what do you want, a boy or a girl?

COSBY: A girl. I don't want any son of mine going through this. (Groans. Fade out.)

Cringe. Maybe the Empathy Belly people were right. But at least this fifties stuff has a wacky integrity and optimism about it. You can also see the play of larger ideas. What I'm watching is how the image of the family and the male role in the family developed during the postwar period. In the fifties and sixties, men, while inept, are at least willing. The humor may come from the idea that these men are often out of their depth, but the point is that they really want to have kids and families. There is also more than a bit of ideology to these shows. *I Love Lucy* had a lot going on under the surface: the dark immigrant sexuality of Ricky Ricardo being transformed and socialized into an American family through the medium of a fair-skinned redhead, Lucille Ball.

Fast forward thirty odd years later, and fatuousness and alienation have replaced the earnestness of *I Love Lucy*. Julie and I recently rented and watched the pre-scandal Hugh Grant in *Nine Months*. It's really a pretty awful film considering that Albert Brooks is the producer. Even I can tell that birthing sequences are total hokum. With real-life situations so full of humor, why does

Hollywood have to invent an inferior simulation? I suppose if I knew the answer to that, I'd be rich and in the film business.

Hugh Grant plays a dithering yuppie shrink with a Porsche, who doesn't want to have children, because he feels that it would limit his career, and *breaks off* his relationship with girlfriend Julianne Moore when he finds out she is pregnant. A further point about men's ambivalence today is made by Jeff Goldblum, who plays Julianne Moore's "struggling artist" brother. (Except that he has a farmhouse in the Napa Valley. I guess that fits the definition of struggle in Beverly Hills.) He goes off on a tirade about the sanctimony of people who have children, when his own artistic contributions should be recognized as worthy and an equivalent contribution to society. So what you're left with is essentially a selfish, effete, male point of view, which is completely alienated from reproduction and family, and is only salvaged by Julianne Moore, another fair-skinned redhead.

The only problem? It's not funny.

If women could, for the nine-month period of their pregnancies, transform themselves and their noncompliant husbands into some other life-form to reproduce, they might consider emperor penguins and sea horses.

I'm lying in the sumptuous luxury of my own personal screening room; that is, I'm propped up on pillows in my bathrobe watching—through my dirty socks—a nature documentary on the pathetic thirteen-inch television at the foot of our bed. Never mind kids, when are we going to get an entertainment center?

Julie's at my side, eating her fourth or fifth Dove bar of the evening. She has turned into a dietary black hole, sucking up all organic matter that isn't nailed down. Julie, from whose dental event horizon no particle of nutrition escapes. I'm actually a little scared. Last week, I was driving back from a day-long business meeting. I was famished, having skipped lunch, and hallucinating about the two shell steaks that were in the fridge, left over from the previous night's dinner party. When I got home they were both gone, as well as everything else in the refrigerator. Julie was there, sitting at the kitchen table with this goofy grin on her face, surrounded by bones and empty cartons. I felt like putting a sign around her neck, "Don't Feed the Bear." I'm actually thinking about caching food around the house. Although in reality I have nothing to worry about. Somehow, after maintaining a weight of 160 pounds since freshman year of college, I've managed to put on seven pounds in four months.

Anyway, nature is not a great place to look for metaphors for fatherhood. In most species it's really a question of males competing among themselves for access to females for sex. In the vast majority of mammals, for example, males have nothing to do with raising offspring. Nature also shows the absolute uselessness of males after insemination by getting rid of them immediately, either by having them die off right away, or in the case of praying mantises and certain spider species, reducing their postcoital value to a caloric level. (Considering Julie's present voraciousness, this may actually be an option.) Then there are all those stories about males actually presenting a danger by eating their young, which were a favorite of my beloved eleventh grade biology teacher.

As this documentary is pointing out, emperor penguins reverse all these stereotypes. While in most penguin species both sexes incubate, in emperor penguins, the males alone perform the incubation duties. After laying their eggs, females leave the colony to head for the shore to feed, often walking fifty to a hundred miles to reach the sea, and do not return until the end of the incubation period, sixty-four days later. Males are left behind through the long

Antarctic winter to incubate and hatch the egg. The male holds the egg on his feet and lives off his stored fat reserves. During violent storms, the males bunch together in tightly packed groups called huddles, for mutual protection from wind and cold.

Sea horse males are even more committed as mates and fathers, actually becoming "pregnant," by carrying the female's eggs in a womblike belly pouch. Once the female develops a clutch of eggs, the male and female perform a reproductive dance, aligning their bodies so that the female can deposit her eggs in the male's pouch. The male releases sperm, fertilizing the eggs internally. A membrane seals the pouch closed, creating a stable environment. A placenta-like organ extends from the pouch wall to handle waste removal and gas exchange while the embryos grow, living off the stored nutrients in the egg. Ten to twelve days later, the father goes into labor, which can last up to two days, releasing a couple of dozen infant sea horses.

Why this high parental-investment strategy on the part of the male? It turns out that while the male is brooding the young, the female is eating as much as possible so she can make a new batch of eggs. (I glance sidelong at Julie, who is keeping her incisors sharpened by gnawing on a box of chocolate chip cookies.) The day after Dad gives birth, Mom returns with the new eggs for fertilization and incubation. This happens over and over again, until over the course of the seven-month breeding cycle, the male is pregnant a dozen times and gives birth to over 300 young. This male investment works to the male's advantage, as it frees up the female to produce as many eggs as possible.

The music swells and the Daddy sea horse's natal sac bursts open. As we marvel at the miniature sea horses streaming upward from the father's belly, I can see Julie getting misty-eyed. Me? I have mixed emotions. Whatever happened to the documentaries of my childhood, such as *Wild Kingdom*, where middle-aged white men roamed the world, tranquilizing everything that moved?

Nature is not what it used to be.

GORDON (driving way too fast down a snowy highway): Can't we keep "Genghis"?

JULIE: No. That's our "womb name." We can't actually name the baby that. Just think what would happen in the schoolyard.

GORDON: All the other kids would be afraid.

JULIE: Great. Besides, what if it's a girl?

GORDON: (now serious): How about Amelia?

JULIE: Too popular.

GORDON: I didn't realize that lost aviatrices were big this year. Emma?

JULIE: Definitely too popular. Jane Austen is huge. Five years from now, half the girls in kindergarten will be named Emma.

GORDON: Eden?

JULIE: Don't you remember? We tried it out on our friends, and everyone hated it. Too weird, too religious.

GORDON: Screw our friends. What do you mean weird? People have been naming children after biblical figures forever. What's wrong with naming her after the actual creation place?

JULIE: I'll think about it. How about Olivia?

GORDON: I can do Olivia.

JULIE: And if it's a boy?

GORDON: Well, I thought that it would be nice to keep the family tradition going and name him Gordon Lee Churchwell the Fourth.

JULIE: That's your family tradition. What about my family? I'm think I'm going to have a problem with this.

GORDON: You don't like my name? You don't want to name our son after me?

JULIE: I love your name. I just think that we need to represent my family somehow. Besides, it's a lot to live up to, being The Fourth. Maybe we can give him a different middle name.

GORDON: But then he wouldn't be Gordon *Lee* Churchwell, the Fourth. He would be something else. And what's so difficult about living up to me? I'm just a poor schlimazel of a writer.

JULIE: How about adding another middle name?

GORDON: What are you suggesting? Gordon Lee Schmuel or Yitzhak Churchwell, the Fourth?

JULIE: Yes, that's exactly what I'm suggesting, except maybe the name would be David or Benjamin.

GORDON: Let me say it again. It wouldn't be the same thing!

JULIE: So what?

GORDON: So what? The whole point of having a tradition like that is to do it *exactly* the same way. Not *kind* of the same way, or *almost* the same way. It either is, or it isn't. Gordon Lee David Churchwell, the Fourth, isn't.

JULIE: I think you're being ridiculous.

GORDON: I'm not being ridiculous. I'm being rational.

JULIE: Fuck you, Mr. Rational. You're driving too fast. You'll get us all killed.

It surprised me, too. Why the obsession with the name thing? I am not exactly someone who is wrapped up in tradition, first of all, and second, what I really want is a girl. Growing up as a boy was so difficult at times—with all those ridiculous rites of passage—that if I had to see a son go through it again, I'm not sure I could bear it. At least with a girl, I wouldn't know what was going on half the time, which is probably better.

So why the outburst? I think I have an answer. I am in the main reading room of the New York Public Library, the most hallowed place for writers in the whole world. Alas, within this shrine to Gutenberg, calfskin, and gold leaf, I sit at a computer station staring at a CRT screen. It's convenient, but feels a little like listening to grunge on your Walkman while touring Beethoven's tomb.

What I'm searching for can hopefully be unlocked with the word "couvade." Couvade means "male childbed," and is derived from *couver*, or "to hatch" in French. The concept is simple, yet hits you like pure magic. A former professor of mine, Edith Kern, turned me on to it. She is sort of like my Obi-Wan Kenobi. As I'm telling her about my little obsession with men and pregnancy, she starts laughing and sends me scurrying off to the library with a tale of this phenomenon among preliterate societies where men engage in pregnancy rituals.

At the time, the story seemed fantastical, yet, appearing on the glowing screen as if by magic, it's coming true. A reference in the *Dictionary of Anthropology*:

Couvade, which refers to the ritual observance by the father of rest and seclusion when his wife gives birth. Commonly both father and mother of the newborn baby must observe certain avoidances relating to food, physical activities, and contact with potentially magically dangerous substances in order to protect the child from harm.

Or the *Encyclopedia of Anthropology*:

Couvade—the imitation by the father of many of the concomitants of childbirth, around the time of his wife's parturition; it is also called "men's childbed." The father may retire to bed, go into seclusion, and observe some taboos and restrictions in order to help the child. Among the theories that have been suggested to account for the *couvade* is that during this period, the father has to take care of himself to avoid an injury that could be transmitted to the child by sympathetic magic. Another is that the father asserts his paternity through appearing to share in the delivery. A third explanation is that the father simulates the wife's activities in order to get evil spirits to focus on him rather than her.

Among the Ainu, the aboriginal people of the northern Japanese islands, "after the delivery the husband joins his wife in postpartum seclusion, where he observes a series of taboos and remains wrapped up near his hearth as if he were ill."

Among the Witoto of the northwestern Amazon, "the husband rests for a week or more in his hammock, observes food taboos, and receives the congratulations of his friends while the new mother is almost ignored."

The Marquesans of Polynesia: "a Marquesan husband takes an active role in the delivery, sometimes holding the mother during the birth."

In the Kurtatchi of Papua New Guinea, the husband secludes himself in a hut nearby while his wife gives birth. "During the delivery and for six days thereafter, he remains in seclusion, ignoring his normal subsistence chores. On the infant's fourth day of life, he makes a medicinal concoction, takes it to the mother and infant, and offers it to the child to make him strong."

Not only is ritual couvade practiced in a great many cultures across the globe, it also has been reported throughout history. "Herodotus lists its existence among certain African tribes. Nymphodorus attributes it to the Scythians at the Black Sea; Diodorus to the Corsicans; Strabo, to the Celto-Iberians of Spain, whose direct descendants, the Basques around the Pyrenees, practice it still. Marco Polo reported the couvade among the mountain tribe of the Miau-tse in his passage to China."

My vision swims as I read on. I feel like Borges deep within the basement of his beloved Beatriz's house, seeing all of history pass before him in the magical sphere of the Aleph. Do so-called preliterate cultures know something we don't? Have men been trying to compensate for their absence of role and control during the birth process since ancient times? Granted, some of the rituals seemed strange and alien, but they also make sense from an emotional point of view. I thought of my recent impulse to impose my surprisingly narrow-minded view of male names.

The number of questions I have are overwhelming, but, for the moment, speaking as a man, I feel as if I have just seen the navel of the world.

> *At the beginning of God's creating*
> *Of the heavens and the earth,*
> *When the earth was wild and waste,*
> *Darkness over the face of the Ocean,*
> *Rushing-spirit of God hovering over the face*
> *of the waters . . .*
> —Everett Fox's translation of Genesis

During their Babylonian exile, the Hebrews found themselves among a people with a capricious pantheon of gods, whose creation myth was violent and terrible. The *Enuma Elish*, the great Babylonian epic, describes how the god Marduk battles and kills Tiamat, the oceanic, primordial goddess. He hews her body in two to form heaven and earth. Humans are then crafted from the bones of Tiamat's lover, the monster Kingu.

Faced with this *X-Men* version of life's beginning, Jewish scholars countered with a creation story of their own, portraying a single omnipotent God, Elohim, who also creates from dark and watery nothingness and chaos, but does it in a structured, logical, and majestic manner. Genesis, from which the world begins perfect, good, and beautiful, is a creation story for a people in need of optimism, affirmation, and control.

The much-dreaded Amnio Day has finally arrived. I'm sitting out in the waiting room, filled, it seems, with equally blank-faced men. Julie is already in the exam room, being prepped for the procedure. It has been a month of anguish for me. As usual, I cannot isolate the exact reason for the way I feel, but I do know instinctively that the amnio carries great symbolic weight. There is the obvious, which is the possibility of having to make a decision about continuing or terminating a life, but at the risk of sounding trite, there's also so much more to it than that.

For my friend David, it took the form of an unacceptable risk: The 0.5 to 1 percent chance of miscarriage was a big deal. This is how he put it: "The doctors and counselors try to tell you that the risk is negligible. It isn't. It's actually pretty high. Think of it this way. What if I told you that if you went outside of your house today, you stood a one in 100 chance of being killed. Would you do it? Of course not. One in a thousand or one in a million, those are odds you don't think about. One in a hundred, or even one in 200? You eat lunch at home."

For Jon, who works for AT&T, it became an obsession with

information: "I needed to know that the baby would be perfect. But there's really no way to guarantee that, is there? The only way to ensure perfection is to test for every possible defect, which is impossible. But I tried anyway. I compulsively pushed my wife, Pat, to take every possible test. It eventually became a big stress point in our relationship. Only now that the baby is here and everything's okay is our life beginning to return to normal."

Then there was the conversation I overheard in an elevator in the Time-Life building. A young secretary is telling her coworker: "My husband is making me get an amnio. I don't see the need. I told him, 'We're not in any risk category . . . I'm twenty-five—don't have to do it.' But he wouldn't stop hounding, so finally I gave in."

And me? I having a real problem with the idea of someone penetrating my wife's body. I know it sounds irrational, but having someone else do it—no matter how expert—goes against the elemental grain. Somehow I've talked myself into the idea that while Dr. Spyros has over twenty years of highly specialized education, training, and experience, it's really me that should be doing this procedure. I guess that's how I know control is one of my big issues.

It's no wonder that men brood over the amniotic waters. Amnio symbolizes a chaotic birthing cosmology. Think of it from the man's perspective. You finally get to participate in the first important decision, and it's all about the potential of a life or death choice, the possibility of literally dismembering your baby. You have to calculate and live with the risk, but the risk isn't taking place in your own body. Nor is there anything you can do to ameliorate it. The only person who can do anything is a complete stranger in whom you have to place absolute trust. It is not a scenario that engenders optimism, affirmation, and control.

A nurse shows me to the ultrasound room. At first all I can

see is the CRT screen with the ultrasound image. After a few seconds, I can make out Julie lying back in a large exam chair. A female ultrasound radiologist is running the transducer over Julie's belly. "One . . . two . . . three . . . four . . . five . . . six . . . seven . . . eight . . . nine . . . ten! And one . . . two . . . three . . . four . . . five . . . six . . . seven . . . eight . . . nine . . . ten! Okay, ten fingers and ten toes. Now, let's take a look between the legs . . . looks like a girl!" Of course everything on the screen is a blur to me. As the radiologist skates the transducer head around, it appears that the fetus is occasionally turning somersaults. How can the radiologist see what she claims to see? And how will Spyros ever get a needle in there without hitting the baby?

Dr. Spyros appears, and suddenly things quiet down. The radiologist searches around and then stabilizes the transducer. She appears to be measuring something. A few more moments, she marks a spot on Julie's belly with a blue pen. Spyros centers the longest needle I have ever seen on the mark, pauses for a moment, and then pushes the needle straight down in one smooth, deliberate motion. On screen, I watch as the needle enters the amniotic sac several centimeters from the fetus's foot. Spyros quickly retracts the plunger, and then smoothly withdraws the needle. The whole procedure has taken less than thirty seconds.

Afterward, we stroll hand in hand up the street to a fancy East Side French bistro to treat ourselves to lunch. With Dr. Spyros's blessing, Julie orders a glass of wine. Soon we're both feeling a little heady, and it's not just the wine, or the bowl of delicious bouillabaisse Julie has ordered, or my plate of sweetbreads. It's the incredible release, and something else . . . her name toddling off our lips. Olivia.

MONTH FIVE

SUBVERSIVE ACTIVITIES

Yet another out-of-body experience. This time, I'm lying on a mat in a studio high above Union Square, pretending to be a woman giving birth. Around me are a dozen couples: The women lie flat on their backs, tilting their pelvises up and down and listening intently to a white unitard-clad instructor; the men look on uncomfortably with dorky expressions. One look at them and it's clear to me that pretending to be a pregnant woman is the less embarrassing option. That's why I'm down with the women, tilting my pelvis with the best of them. Plus what choice do I really have? Seeing the look of epic determination on Julie's face as she tries to build up her abdominals into a baby howitzer, I realize that all this intensity can lead to only one option: Get with the program or receive a beating.

So I'm down on the mat tilting and squeezing. Our instructor stalks among us, barking out commands. Her unitard makes her look like a refugee from *Logan's Run* or some other sci-fi utopia-gone-wrong movie of the 1970s. Her manner, however, is all Lee Marvin in *The Dirty Dozen*:

"Okay, ladies, there's no turning back! So long as you are going to be there, you might as well be strong and empowered. You need to start training for your birth early in your pregnancy. You wouldn't run a marathon without training for it, would you? Pregnancy is the same thing. It's an athletic event, a race that you can't pull out of. You need to get those pushing muscles in shape. You also need to learn about nutrition; later I'll teach you about carbo-loading. And you need to get that mind/body connection established."

There's nothing a man loves more in a metaphor than sports, except perhaps war, but hearing this, I'm skeptical. Somehow visualizing these women—galumphing around on flat feet, groaning and holding their backs, having to urinate every five seconds—as Olympic athletes is beyond my powers.

As if she's reading my mind, the instructor looks directly at me. "And your husbands need to get involved!" She continues, scanning us male recruits with a novel combination of compassion and disgust, "It's not okay for the men to hold your hand and say, 'Breathe, honey.' You need someone there to be your advocate and to know what you want."

Next we're on all fours. "All the action starts from the pubic bone. You know what that action is, don't you, ladies, or else you wouldn't be here in this condition!"

You might think that seeing ten women on all fours in the doggie position tilting and thrusting their pelvises would be erotic. Instead, it looks more like a roomful of cats coughing up hairballs in unison. Apparently this motion also places considerable pressure on the bladder, for soon there is a trickle, and then a stream of women excusing themselves to go to the bathroom.

Exercise programs for pregnant women arose because childbirth educators realized there was a void to fill. These programs are founded on two breathtakingly simple ideas: (1) A women should be in optimal physical condition for her labor and delivery, training the specific muscles so that she can have more control over the process. (2) Childbirth education should start early in pregnancy, not at the end, as is conventionally done.

Now, the instructor has got us on our backs again, attempting a dry run of what she calls "the squeeze." The theory sounds elegant and fundamentally sound. Practice the activity you are going to do. Build up your abdominal muscles so that when it comes time to push, you can exert pressure on the uterus and help push the baby down and out of the birth canal. What separates this technique from traditional pushing is that force is applied not by holding your breath and bearing down, but with exhalation, as in yogic breathing.

"The innermost abdominal is my favorite muscle, that's the transverse muscle. It's like a corset. This is the muscle that pushes your baby out. Think of pushing that baby out like squeezing toothpaste out of the tube. Now, squeeeeze! But don't hold your breath! Why don't you hold your breath? Because then you can't get any oxygen! No O_2! Plus you might get popped blood vessels in your eyes. And worst case, you've all heard of ladies having strokes during labor, haven't you? So why in the middle of labor do the nurses tell you to bear down? Because it's an easy thing to say and an easy thing to do. You need to practice my technique. This is not something you can do if you don't practice. When is the best time to practice? When you're having a bowel movement. Having a baby is like having a bowel movement—the biggest and best you've ever had. Okay, squeeeeze!"

In my zeal to mimic their actions, I suddenly realize that I've taken the pushing and squeezing too far. Something down there is heading for the exit, and I'm just moments away from defecating on the mat.

Luckily, "the squeeze" is reversible, and soon we're on to the next lecture-cize. "I want you to do at least five sets of 100 kegels every day! That's 500 repetitions! This is your best chance of avoiding an episiotomy. You need to build up your pelvic floor so that your perineum is strong and supple. Doctors will tell you that a strong perineum makes birthing more difficult. They're wrong! A strong muscle is a stretchy muscle! The stronger it is, the suppler it is; the more it will be able to stretch and bounce back. Husbands take note! The stronger your wife's perineum, the sooner you'll be able to have sex after the delivery. If your wife has an episiotomy . . . it could be months. So make sure she does her kegels!"

Ah, yes, the sex carrot. Just in case my male brain couldn't grasp the point.

We take a break and some handouts are passed around. The first couple of pages are descriptions of exercises. Then comes a sheet titled "The Philosophy of Birth," which contains statements such as:

"The knowledge to give birth is within each woman."

"Women and babies are designed to give birth and to be born safely."

"Birth is a normal process that doesn't require tools, machines, or chemicals."

"Having accomplished a natural birth, there is nothing in the world a woman cannot do!"

What does it mean? The list is about as compelling as an eye chart. I read it twice, trying to get the words to sink in. This thing must come from the same Hallmark Card School of Existentialism that produces those crocheted lists of platitudes that hang in dentists' offices with titles like "Love Is . . ." and serve to provoke, in me, barely resistible impulses toward serial murder.

The last handout stops me. It's a reprint from a magazine

with the title "The Unkindest Cut?" which appears in large type just below an even larger photograph of a pair of gleaming stainless steel surgical shears. The subtitle reads: "Episiotomy is performed in nearly half of all vaginal births—a figure that experts agree probably is too high."

The article goes on to describe how many obstetricians will enlarge a woman's vaginal opening as she is giving birth, by making an incision with a scalpel or surgical scissors through part of the perineum, from the lower edge of the vagina toward the anus. It's a technique meant to be used in certain complicated deliveries: to speed delivery when the baby is in distress; to ease breech births; to create room for forceps; or when the vaginal opening is too tight to pass the baby's head without tearing, especially tearing toward the front of the vagina (an injury that is particularly difficult and painful to recuperate from).

The point of the article seems to be that despite the fact that episiotomies have scientifically proven benefits in only a limited number of situations, and are not recommended as standard practice by the American College of Obstetricians and Gynecologists, many OBs employ the technique routinely. Half of the women delivering in the United States receive episiotomies, the majority of these cases being first deliveries. The consequences for women? Episiotomies, according to the article, worsen rather than prevent tearing, are painful to recover from, occasionally lead to infection, and diminish the perineum's ability to stretch in future.

"Okay, ladies, episiotomy is my special thing and I'm going to tell you how you're going to talk about it with your doctor. Don't say, 'I don't want to have an episiotomy.' You'll only piss your doctor off and the wall will go up. Doctors only listen to other doctors. What you have to do is say, 'So, how do you feel about episiotomies?' Your doctor will, of course, say, 'I only do them if necessary.' But that's not enough. Everyone is going to say that. What you have to find out is what their attitudes are toward first-time mothers. You need to ask, 'For a first-time mom, how often do you think an episiotomy is necessary?' If your doctor says 1 percent, you know you're in the presence of an enlightened being. If your doctor says 50 percent, you know you're going to get one. Anything under 10 percent . . . it's a good place to start. Remember, ladies, your birth is not a technological event! You need to know if your OB feels the same way. If not, you need to find out sooner rather than later, so you can make a choice to go with your present doctor or find a new one."

My head is swimming. Find a new doctor? Technological event? What is all this fuss about what seems to be a very simple and not overly invasive procedure?

At this point, Lee Marvin starts in again. "And men, you need to be the Fetus Police! Read *The Birth Partner*. You need to be an informed advocate for your partner. When she's in the middle of pushing she won't be able to negotiate for herself. So, you need to know what she wants out of her birth, and you have to be able to help her get it. Okay, any questions?"

Every woman's hand shoots up. As I survey the women's faces, including the face of my Julie, grim and intent, it's clear that I—and, judging from their stunned and hapless expressions, all the other men—have been missing something, something big.

Insurrection is in the air.

It's not like she told me all at once. "Oh, by the way honey, I'm having a natural birth." On the other hand, it wasn't like I was paying attention, either.

Now that I think of it, I seem to recall that along with those books with the horrible pictures of women squatting somewhere in Scandinavia, there was also a running commentary about how interested she was, how much sense natural delivery made. That was the part I blocked out completely. There was no way I could imagine my Julie giving birth like that, and besides, that's not how we do it in America. In America, women lie on their backs in a hospital delivery room emitting an occasional moan and whimper, which are soon soothed with drugs I only dreamed about in college. Doctors, cheered on by a phalanx of nurses and interns, and backed by an armamentarium of technologies appropriate to the richest country on the planet, then issue stern exhortations to push, or else. Moments later, after one, no maybe two sharp cries from the moms, the babies arrive, healthy, alert, and ready for their first cereal commercial. That's how it's done in America. I know; I've seen it a hundred times on television.

Julie, on the other hand, keeps talking to me about the "quality of the experience." Her desire to "have her *own* experience." To be in "control of *her* experience." So much so that I'm beginning to wonder whether childbirth education is actually a hidden form of EST seminars for pregnant women.

This really irritates me. Julie billed the pregnancy exercise program as getting in shape for pregnancy, not a guerrilla movement. After all, our friend Miranda recommended it to us, and she is about as hard-nosed as they come: Smith, B.A.; Harvard, M.B.A.; management consultant. Nothing crunchy-granola about her. Besides our own OB wrote one of the brochure blurbs for the program.

What is a "natural" birth anyway? Is Julie going to slink off into the woods to have a baby? Does that mean having a baby at home? Who but an insane person would want to have a baby at home, instead of a hospital? Who would want someone other than a doctor in attendance performing the delivery? Who would want to take those risks, and for what conceivable purpose? Specifically, why would Julie want to take this kind of risk with our firstborn?

And why the fear of technology? I have personally seen doctors save the lives of babies that weigh 900 grams, taking up no more room than a sparrow in the palm of your hand, their limbs practically transparent when held up to the light. Surely, if doctors can deliver and sustain such a baby, a normal delivery should be child's play.

I have to admit that I am more than a little angry at the situation. All my life I have loved and believed in technology. I can remember as a kid waiting for Dad's monthly subscription of *Popular Science* to arrive, marveling endlessly at notions such as flying cars. My favorite books were those about Tom Swift and by Jules Verne. Everything seemed to fly, levitate on a cushion of air. Everything was convenient, instantaneous, and flawless. Slow nature seemed irrelevant.

The ultimate fantasy, of course, was the domed city, a city of the future where people lived happy lives in an environment that was safe, no matter where the domed city was, whether in the middle of the desert, on the ocean floor, or on Mars. No matter where this city was, inside all the needs of the people were cared for with technology and automation. It was a vision that was strangely womblike, and the women of this city?

They did not squat to give birth.

Childbirth educators want you to be, above all, "informed consumers" capable of making the best possible choices for yourself. If only it were that simple.

On the surface, birth seems to be a continuum of choices. On one end is walking into the hospital and asking for Demerol at the admissions desk on your way to your scheduled C-section. The other is having your baby at home, surrounded by a chorus of midwife shamans singing "'Tis a gift to be simple" *a cappella* as you squat on your haunches and howl with pain. If you're smart, somewhere in between, is your birth.

The idea that birth is a continuum or spectrum and that there is consumer choice is a bit of an illusion. In reality almost all births in the United States take place in the hospital under the care of obstetricians. Even if a midwife attends you, doctors are in charge. Contrast this to many European countries where large numbers of births take place at home or in birthing centers, and are primarily managed by midwives, with OBs as auxiliaries.

What makes birth in America so difficult for expecting couples is the conflicted soul of American reproduction. The truth is that midwives, labor nurses, childbirth educators, and OBs work side-by-side in the United States, but by no means are their thoughts on the same page. In fact, there is a profound internal conflict in philosophy, policy, and practice. This is highly disconcerting to birth novitiates. After all, with all the potentially warm and fuzzy feelings surrounding birth and babies, with all the money to be made from expecting parents gone ga-ga, with all the anxiety that needs to be quelled, what you'd expect to encounter is a birth industry with its shit together, something typically American, with all the pathological attention to detail and consumer coddling of a company like Disney. Instead, what you get is a DMZ in a cultural war that comes complete with propaganda, infiltration, collaborators, and surgical strikes.

Somewhere in here is a Vietnam metaphor. The natural birth cadres are winning the hearts and minds of pregnant women, but the doctors control the hospitals.

What pisses me off about all this is that, in addition to all my own demons, I have to deal with a birth industry that engenders and provokes doubt and anxiety, rather than alleviates it. All of a sudden I am asked to question the philosophy and practice of our doctor. Secondly, I now not only have to worry about Julie's health, I have to worry about the quality of her experience, and the quality of her intentions. Is her zeal to have a "natural delivery," to fulfill some feminist destiny, going to put our baby's health at risk? Look, all I want to do is have a baby, safe and sound, not make a political statement or weigh in on a centuries-old debate.

It's amazing how far apart the two camps can be. Half the people who are supposed to be helping you are hawking the virtues of natural birth and telling you that you're about to be operated on by the Evil Empire, while the other half is threatening you with visions of what could happen to your fetus if you don't have the latest gizmo handy, just in case.

First, the midwives' point of view.

In the beginning . . .

Midwives tend to speak with one voice, and the tale goes something like this:

Women's bodies were designed by nature to give birth. Since the beginning of what we know of as human life, women have given birth naturally with the support of other women. At some point, this support system was institutionalized in the existence of the midwife.

For midwives, pregnancy and birth is a unique physiological and psychological experience and process for each woman. They believe that the woman's emotional state during pregnancy and childbirth is perhaps the preeminent driver of the birth process. Many midwives feel in their hearts that home deliveries are the ideal, closely followed by freestanding birth centers. In these environments—free from the alien environment and restrictive practices of the hospital, free from the electronic monitors, analgesics, rules against eating, and a twelve-hour labor time limit—a second radical idea is born.

Supported and at ease, a birthing woman becomes the author of the birth. She is free to choose: to move around, to try different positions, to sit in the tub, and eat to keep her strength up. She is free to enjoy the company of her loved ones, free to accept the advice of her chosen, expert birth attendants. Free to take six, twelve, eighteen, twenty-four, thirty-six, or more hours to birth her baby.

And what of pain? She is free to accept pain as part of the process of birth. Pain becomes a sort of internal guidance system. Pain lets you know that you need to shift positions, to help ameliorate the pain, and in doing so, help the delivery along. Pain is both rational knowledge and initiation into the mysteries of self—a psychic marker, an inner tattoo, a signatory in one's personal myth, and most important, a future source of power.

Then came the Fall . . .

Evil came into the picture when men became involved in birth, encroaching on women's natural territory, somewhere around the late 1700s in the form of surgeon/barbers—who subsequently evolved into what we know as doctor/obstetricians. Men brought interventional techniques into birth, such as the forceps, and a mechanistic view. Eventually, men forced midwives out of business by redefining expertise in birth as interventional, casting doubt on the skills of midwives, and using their growing political and cultural power to restrict midwives' access to the marketplace.

Next came gender politics . . .

Men's involvement in birth has been a steady process of colonization of women's bodies. Men are afraid of the sexual power of women, and have no way of understanding the experience of what it means to be a woman and what it means to give birth. So men try to exert control and power over women by "managing" the birth process using technological aids and interventions that give them access and control over women's bodies. Men have taken control of birth as a way of consolidating cultural power over women.

The struggle between Good and the American Medical Association . . .

As in all great metaphysical debates, there are two very different versions of reality.

The Death Star of American birth is the active management model. Obstetricians, according to midwives, practice a "disease model" of pregnancy, viewing pregnancy as a pathological state. I've never been able to fully understand this analogy, but what I think midwives mean is that obstetricians see birth as inherently risky and imperfect process, and as a threat to the mother. They see women's bodies as a less than ideal place to have reproduction take place. They set about to reduce the risk by throwing technologies and interventions at it. This "active management" model of birth was actually invented in the early 1970s at the National Maternity Hospital in Dublin, Ireland. American OBs then brought the idea across the pond and souped it up for the U.S. market.

This is the way it's supposed to work:

1: You call your OB groaning with pain at regular intervals. The OB makes a diagnosis of labor based on painful contractions combined with full effacement of the cervix, and/or rupture of the membranes.

2: One hour after admission, your OB assesses your progress. If the membranes haven't ruptured, the OB performs an amniotomy, or ruptures the membranes.

3: Your cervix must dilate by at least one centimeter per hour. Otherwise, labor is augmented by giving you an pitocin IV drip, until you experience five to seven contractions every fifteen minutes.

4: Meanwhile, the doctor keeps tabs on your baby's heartbeat with continuous electronic fetal monitoring (EFM) . . .

5: And to help you with your pain, you can start out with Demerol and move on to an epidural.

You're also on a schedule. Maximum labor length is twelve hours—ten hours to dilate, two hours to push the baby out. More time, and the possibility of infection increases, or so the reasoning goes.

So what is wrong with this system that produces a 1.1 percent infant mortality rate?

What modern metaphysical debate would be complete without statistics?

The way it is implemented in the United States, active management throws off a 25 percent C-section rate, ranking the United States third in the world, behind Puerto Rico and Brazil—that's one out of every four women having C-sections. Secondly, we habitually rank low in terms of infant mortality among Western industrialized nations—try twenty-first in the world. So what is it about our high-tech method of giving birth that creates risk and promotes such high rates of intervention?

As in all great moral debates, there is a "slippery slope" argument . . .

The 800-pound gorilla of labor and delivery problems is the dreaded labor dystocia or "failure to progress," meaning that labor is not proceeding or proceeding too slowly given the twelve-hour time window. OBs feel that labors which proceed beyond this time limit incur risks of fetal infection and fetal distress, making labor dystocia one of the leading rationales for cesarean.

Midwives argue that the active management model is a cascading sequence of interventions and missteps that in fact cause labor dystocia. Since midwives proceed from the point of view that birth is a natural process, their first criticism of the active management program is that it starts out in an unnatural environment. You feel contractions, you call your OB. He or she listens to you whine on the phone and then calls you in to the hospital for a cervical exam. So, at the very beginning of labor, you find yourself in a strange and unpleasant environment, surrounded by strangers, having your crotch felt up. You feel uncomfortable and anxious, so—like primates who have been known to stop labor and go into hiding when they are observed—your labor stops or slows down.

An hour later when they check you again and you're not dilating sufficiently, you'll get "pitted," or receive an IV drip of pitocin. Since pitocin increases the strength of contractions, it also increases the possibility of fetal distress. So if you haven't been wired up yet by now, you receive continuous electronic fetal monitoring, meaning you wear a belt with electrodes. Wearing this thing, along with the IV, further inhibits your movements, so any ideas you had about using your body to help your own labor and delivery—say walking around or moving from position to position—just became significantly more difficult. Stronger contractions also mean more pain, which means an epidural. The epidural anesthesia further retards labor, and when it comes time to push, makes pushing very, very difficult, if not impossible.

Add to this other details such that most OBs still use the lithotomy position for delivery. This is the classic woman-on-her-back, OB-peering-into-her-vagina position that does nothing to promote a successful delivery. With the lithotomy position the pelvis is actually tilted upward, requiring the baby to travel "uphill" at the end. As one midwife put it, "Where's the gravity?" The final insult is that if you actually make it to a vaginal birth you stand perhaps an 80 percent chance of having an unnecessary episiotomy.

So there you have it-a self-fulfilling prophecy as paradigm. The active management model sees a lot of women with labor dystocia requiring intervention because the active management of labor—with its hospital environment, pitocin drips, epidural sticks, electronic fetal monitoring, and artificial time constraints—actually causes labor dystocia. Or to put it another way, it sees a lot of women with failure to progress because it fails to allow them to progress and thus creates the need to intervene.

Beyond the paradigm, there's the metaphor . . .

In case you didn't realize what was at stake, many midwives think that the way the conventional medical establishment handles birth says something about the way our society values life.

One midwife I spoke to said it this way: "It's much larger than just a feminist issue. It speaks to Western culture and how little we value our individuals as people, as employees, as fathers, as mothers, as children, as families. We don't support our humanity in this country. We don't honor the postpartum period in any way. We take discharge time and make it into a clinical issue, as if the forty-eight hours of mandated hospital time addresses the critical six-week postpartum period, or addresses the lack of education the mother has moving into this new world. How we see birth is just part of a larger diseased state with our country."

"Squeeze the baby out like toothpaste, huh? Well I've got news for you. That would be fine if the baby was as malleable as toothpaste, but the baby isn't toothpaste."

Allan, an OB/GYN with a Park Avenue practice, is giving me the other side of the birth story. Allan is not the Prince of Darkness. He's a nice Jewish boy who's made good, and a happy man—happy in life and happy in his work. And why shouldn't he be? He's got almost as much walnut paneling in his office as the *Titanic*.

I have to say that waiting for him in his waiting room, I noted several things. There were no men. Many of the women who were waiting were obviously very wealthy. There was enough Prada and Chanel to start a boutique. Perhaps half the women seemed to have utilized some form of plastic surgery. One woman had the complexion of a trampoline. After about forty-five minutes of studying them, I came to the unassailable conclusion that none of these women had squatted to give birth.

When I tell him about the article "The Unkindest Cut?" he goes ballistic.

"'The Unkindest Cut' is unfair. It's shrill, it's polarizing, and it's just not true. There's no question that doctors do too many episiotomies, and both doctors and patients should be politicized about the issue. But it's ultimately a matter of judgment, and being against too many episiotomies doesn't end the issue of the need for episiotomies in a significant number of cases, and the artfulness of the doctor in making the judgment, and then performing the procedure in a way that achieves the best possible outcome.

"This is a woman's vagina," he said, leaning forward in his armchair and cupping his left hand into a circle. "This is the baby," forcing his right fist through the aperture. "Remember what I said about the baby not being toothpaste? The baby goes through this opening that doesn't stretch that much." He forced his right fist through the vessel formed by his left hand. Soon, his fingers gave way.

"I think the worst mistake you can make is not to do an episiotomy when you should have, because then the patient suffers and you, meaning the doctor, are not happy, because you have a ragged tear on your hands. Even though it sounds terribly old-fashioned, an episiotomy is neat, and it saves the urethra, the clitoris, and the labia from ripping and being damaged. On the other hand, it does hurt a little afterwards, and it does increase the possibility of injury to the anus and rectum."

What about the claim that episiotomies can actually increase tearing?

Let's talk about that. There are two things midwives like to do. First, they like to say that they can avoid episiotomies and that they only have to sew a little bit. That's true to some extent. Yes, in some cases if you massage a tremendous amount over a long period of time, you can ultimately stretch out the vagina and get only a little bit of tearing.

The other thing they do is lie. Their patients tear more

than they say they tear. They call a severe tear a moderate tear, a moderate tear a mild tear, and a mild tear a trifle. I'm convinced they exaggerate their results. It's true that you get more anal injury with an episiotomy than without, but my answer to that is 'Let's look at the vagina that saved that rectum.' If that's what a vagina looks like after all the ripping and tearing, I say to hell with it. Make a wee cut, even if it extends toward the rectum, and protect the vagina. Afterwards, you can sew them back together again.

So let's move on to bigger game. What about the historical claim that doctors screwed things up by introducing intervention into childbirth?

That's the product of a romantic view of history, and I find no romance in the past, medically speaking. Speaking about the bulk of history, there's no romance in a life expectancy of thirty to thirty-five years. Did you know that life expectancy didn't pass fifty until 1900? As for birth, half the babies died. Half. And did you know that in the America of the 1930s one in 200 mothers died in childbirth? So much for the romance of the past.

What about the claim that doctors colonized childbirth, kicking out the midwives?

Look, first of all, I want you to know that I have nothing against midwives. The reason I know about these issues at all is that the type of informed patient who might consider a midwife might also be in my practice. I have a reputation for practicing humanely. My heroes include a doctor who delivered patients in bed and had the fathers cut the umbilical cord back in 1976. My partner, who is a woman, and I grew up emulating his practice and individualizing our approach to our patients. So we birthed woman in beds before there were 'birthing beds,' and we let fathers cut umbilical cords before it was fashionable. We have a style of delivery that is simpatico with many of the things midwives believe in, and I'm somewhat of a centrist on many of the issues we're talking about.

Having said that, there was no "Golden Age" of midwifery or childbirth. They were in the same boat as everyone else. Midwives didn't have any better ways of dealing with crises in pregnancies than doctors. Did they wash their hands and doctors didn't? No. Did they have penicillin before it was discovered? Did they have modern techniques for dealing with hemorrhage? Did they deal with childbed fever any better? No.

The truth is what we have now is a luxury. As the death rate of babies has gone down, as the death rate of mothers has gone down, the political sensitivity of women has been in ascendancy. People wake up and say, "You know what? This could stand a little correction."

So what you're saying is that birth is naturally a risky process . . .

Nature without medical progress is desperately unsuccessful from a twenty-first-century yuppie point of view. Do you think nature requires 100 percent results? Fifty percent survival will do just fine. Do you think nature requires people with higher IQs? Evolution doesn't require a 140 IQ. You just need people to stay alive and reproduce. Prehistoric men and women, if they knew anything intellectually, knew it was a crap shoot when it came to birth. Cave Guy was sweating it out, wondering whether, when it was all over, he would have both his mate and his child. That's nature, and as long as each set of parents had more than two children, the population would remain stable or grow. That's all nature cares about.

And it was only the development of interventions that made it safer?

In a very short time the development of our intellects and of our societies have led us into an unnatural set of expectations. Remember, I told you that in 1935 one in 200 mothers died in childbirth. Do you think that is risky?

Yes.

Well, by 1945 it was one in 1,000. And now we have ratcheted it down to one in 10,000. How did that happen? I admit we surgerized obstetrics, we surgerized delivery. We shaved the mother. We tied the mother down and anesthetized the mother. We discovered fetal monitoring and did cesarean sections for every little blip. We screwed up, but not in an arrogant way. We did it in good faith. We screwed up in a "young, scared, want-to-do-well-for-the-mother-and-patient" way. We had to learn. But we also accomplished something. We went from one in 200 maternal deaths in 1935 to one in 1,000 in 1945, to one in 10,000 now. That's a five-fold, and then a fifty-fold advancement. That was pro-woman, pro-baby, pro-health advancement, and it was accomplished through technology.

Now that we've accomplished all this advancement, now we can return in an artful, humane, manner to dress up medical progress. We're humanizing the surroundings and the circumstances. We're doing it with the mother awake. We're inviting the father to come in and participate. The grandparents can come in and say hello. We can add all of the wonderful human warmth to the process, but still keep every bit of medical progress.

What about the claim that the midwifery model involves minimal intervention, preserves the autonomy of the mother, and is just as good?

Like I said, I have nothing against midwives. I have no reason to deny them credibility—they're doing good work with a good level of science. I've no reason to not listen to what they have to say. Frankly the literature on the fact that you can save the rectum by not doing an episiotomy was midwife-driven stuff. I don't quite know what to do with it, because it leads you into some artful conflicts, but I listen to what they come up with.

But you have to understand that it's just not that pure out there. Midwives have their problems, too. There are some midwives who get a little quirky and let the mother push for five hours and try eight different position, when it would be clear to a reasonable midwife practitioner that this kid wasn't coming out without help. The heart rate is ninety, there's meconium* all over the place, and the kid is in trouble. A doctor would diagnose fetal distress. I mean, get the kid out of there!

So midwives, like doctors, sometimes take themselves and their politics and their preferences a little too seriously. Along with the Western sins of too many episiotomies, there are Eastern sins, too.

---

*Meconium is the baby's own waste product that builds up during the pregnancy. It is usually jettisoned after birth in the baby's first bowel movement. Meconium during delivery is a sign of fetal distress.

Midwives would argue that C-sections are also responsible for higher infant mortality. Combine pitocin and epidurals with fetal monitoring and you have a recipe for inappropriate cesareans. The drugs go in, the monitor dives, you guys jump in with knives flashing.

Yes. I'm not going to be a fool and argue that cesareans are as safe as vaginal deliveries, although I will say that there was one study done in Boston that had 10,000 C-sections in a row without one death.

A midwife would say, wait on the mother, and use auscultation* instead of monitoring. Studies have shown that auscultation is—

Let me tell you something about auscultation. It's political. I was recently at a meeting of some medical school professors. They were coming out with a consensus statement for publication. They talked about fetal monitoring and how it could lead to too many C-sections, which is true. But the issue has its subtler side. So I said, "If you're talking about subtle things on the monitor that are important but are being missed by auscultation, why don't you come out against it?" They said, "We think auscultation sucks, but we're afraid the editors wouldn't publish us if we said it." So they weren't willing to take the political heat. They didn't want to piss off the midwife establishment and start some fatwah, and they were afraid that the editors, of the obstetrics journal mind you, wouldn't publish them.

---

*Auscultation is listening to the fetal heartbeat with the stethoscope pressed against the mother's abdomen.

What about the studies that show that auscultation and fetal monitoring are equivalent?

It depends on what you're measuring. If you measure cerebral palsy you may not be able to tell the difference between monitoring and auscultation. But if you measure for something subtler, like IQ, who knows? There's a study done in the Israeli military that shows that the longer the labor the lower the IQ. It was the simplest study. Everyone has to get an IQ test at eighteen. So you take the test result, correlate it with the length of labor from the medical chart, and hand it to a computer. The longer labors had lower IQs and the shorter labors had higher IQs.

My head reeled. I thought about some of those women in the waiting room, their faces stretched like tambourines. So that's how their sons and daughters got into Yale and Princeton—Mom's selfless embrace of intervention in all its forms.

So let me try to paraphrase here without loading the dice. What you're saying is that birth is inherently risky. We haven't even gotten to the point yet when we can accurately measure some of the deficits caused by the natural birth process. So when midwives say, look at these studies—

The probes have been too coarse.

Our measurements aren't fine enough?

Exactly. There's a hint from some of the studies that you really can't trust labor that much. Labor may be natural, but it's not harmless. We don't have the tests yet which can adequately measure the differences, especially because of all of the sociocultural diversity in America. But the danger is that we may never find out because of the political contamination. Think of the incredible modern irony. You have doctors, professors of medicine, suppressing legitimate opinion because they don't want to piss off midwives and others in the anti-doctor community.

I would also like to point out another irony. Here you are defending the preservation of . . . I don't know how many IQ points you have in mind, by saying that we don't yet have the tools necessary to measure them. . . . Doesn't that suggest that the deficits may be very slight indeed?

I'm not trying to defend cesarean sections. I'm just saying stop with the auscultation stuff already. I am for judicious judgment. Women have to have faith. They have to trust that the system we have really works, and thank goodness old-fashioned "trust your doctor" is still winning, and I don't think it will ever go away.

Doctors, in turn, need to be worthy of that trust. We don't have all of the answers. We're going to know things in twenty years we don't know now. But I'll take the imperfection of a doctor acting in good faith over the politicized person who goes back and says, "I think childbirth is very safe." That's bad faith, bad history, bad scholarship, bad integrity, bad everything. I'll take my awkwardness, my impurity, my well-meant, well-read imperfection over somebody whose opening statement is "The world of OBs is all screwed up. Pitocin is bad. Epidurals are bad. Don't trust this outfit." I think the poor son-of-a-bitch who's in there thinking, critically evaluating, dancing as fast as he can is more worthy of respect than the shrill critics who take their politics as their first agenda. Their agenda is not the mother and the baby, it's espousing their egos. Their happiness lies in their vanity, not in good health practice.

As I walked out the door past those women sitting patiently behind their carefully constructed smiles, I could not have agreed more.

GORDON: Listen to this. A Brooklyn jury awarded $45 million to a girl who suffered brain damage after doctors gave her mother too much anesthesia during childbirth. The girl is twelve now and still suffers from cerebral palsy.

JULIE: That's horrible. Pass the eggs, and make another pot of herbal tea, would you?

(Later that evening.)

GORDON: How long was Willow in labor?

JULIE: Three days.

GORDON: First delivery?

JULIE: Yeah, she tried for a home birth on her first delivery.

GORDON: And the midwife waited three days before getting her to a hospital? She ended up with a C-section, right?

JULIE: Three days at home in the middle of a snowstorm before going for help. But at least everything worked out for Willow. Her neighbor wasn't as lucky. She had the same thing happen to her, but her baby had something wrong with him.

GORDON: They sure do things differently in Vermont. What were they thinking?

Our new sport consists of sitting at the kitchen table, reading each other news items about births gone bad. Or sitting in bed at night, remembering stories about friends of friends who had bad birthing experiences. It's not because we're morbid or masochists. In fact, it's just the opposite. We alternately seem to be suffering from some sort of information hypoxia, where our little brains are desperately trying to extract enough information out of thin air to make us feel more comfortable about the decisions we're about to make. Then, at other times, it seems we're drowning in it.

Making decisions without enough information is a time-honored tradition. Most of us have plenty of strategies to allow ourselves to act, or not to act, without the benefit of knowing too much or anything at all. Which works fine most of the time except when you are faced with a situation where there is really no escape. Once you are pregnant, like it or not, something is going to happen to you, and most of us harbor anxieties that that something or—placed in the context of the obstetrician-midwife debate—someone could possibly harm or kill you and/or your baby.

Anxiety or the perception of danger heightens your senses. A year ago, an article about childbirth would never have made it onto our radar screens. Now, over scrambled eggs, toast, and the hateful tea, it seems that all the issues we've been pondering for the last five months are also being played out in the society around us.

One day brings news of a $45 million court judgment against a hospital; another brings a report of a midwife having her license suspended for allowing a patient to endure thirty hours of labor at home, even though the patient's cervix had barely dilated. The midwife did not consult her backup physician, and left the patient's house several times. The baby died from inhaling meconium after sixty-eight hours of labor.

In this kind of environment how can you make an intelligent decision about your own pregnancy? Whom can you trust? Who's telling the truth? About history? About nature? Are women marvels of nature? Or imperfect organic machines, with an unacceptable quality control rate to suit the needs of modern culture, and in need of constant supervision and adjustment?

Looking into the history of childbirth, one is immediately struck by how complex the issues really are, and how consistent the themes have been.

First, some history.

Midwives and obstetricians have been going at it not just for decades but for centuries. Catherine Schrader, a Dutch midwife in the early 1700s, complained that "male physicians who attended birth were too rough and too crude, too ready to pronounce the baby dead when it failed to suck on a finger, too ready to lop off limbs when the labor was an abnormal presentation . . ."

Prior to this point, midwives had birthing duties pretty much all to themselves. An excerpt from Soranus's *Gynaecology* provides instructions for the first-century Roman midwife.

> For normal childbirth have the following ready: oil for injections and cleansing, hot water in order to wash the affected area, hot compresses to relieve the labour pains, sponges for sponging oft; a birthing stool so that the mother may be arranged on it . . .

The character of birth was completely different from what we know now. Birth undertaken alone and in isolation was viewed with extreme suspicion. It was a communal experience, village theater, with the laboring woman being attended by midwives and a crowd of female relatives, friends, and neighbors. Midwives held a valued if ambiguous place in society. In early America, they were often place on "retainer," that is, given free housing in return for being available to the community. While at times viewed by suspicion by the clergy, in Catholic countries midwives were empowered to perform emergency baptisms on infants who died in childbirth.

Was there a golden age of midwifery?

No. There was a reason women wanted as much support, companionship, and counsel around them as possible. Childbirth was a grim business. More than 20 percent of children died before their first birthday in eighteenth-century Europe. Five percent of newborns died during birth or from some birth-related trauma or infection.

The odds for mothers were equally grim. Death could come in a great variety of forms, hemorrhage and infection being the greatest killers. A woman's ability to withstand the stresses of childbirth or to give birth without complications was often compromised by health problems such as tuberculosis and sexually transmitted diseases, or nutritional problems such as rickets, which caused malformation of the pelvis. Judith Walzer Leavitt, in her *Brought to Bed: Childbearing in America, 1750–1950*,* provides a thorough and balanced account of the conditions that women faced throughout the history of childbirth in the United States.

Looking at a relatively modern standard, 1910, by which time statistics had improved considerably over earlier standards, a woman stood a more than one in 150 chance of dying during childbirth. Consider that the average woman delivered five children, the risk compounded to a one in thirty chance of dying during a woman's childbearing years. In an early twentieth-century

*Oxford University Press, 1986.

study, one in seventeen men who applied for life insurance revealed that he had a mother or sister who had died as the immediate result of childbirth.

Death from childbirth, however, was only the beginning of a woman's problems. Childbirth often inflicted long-term and permanent disability. The lacerations that midwives and obstetricians joust over today in prior centuries could prove lethal. Women suffered from tears in the perineum or in the walls of the vagina, bladder, and rectum. In the worst cases, the violence of birth or instruments could cause fistulas to form—holes between the vagina and bladder or rectum that allow urine or feces to leak into the vagina. Another frequent problem was a prolapsed uterus, or "fallen womb," where the uterus was displaced downward, sometimes through the vagina, as a result of lacerations and the weakening of ligaments in the pelvic floor.

The fear that childbirth caused in women was perhaps even more profound than the statistics. Given that most women's lives were devoted to childbearing soon after marriage, given that the lack of effective contraception meant that a woman was continually trapped in the reproductive cycle—pregnant, giving birth, recovering from birth, getting pregnant again—given that the average woman had five children or more, life must have seemed like a constant dice-shoot with death. In an absolute sense, women spent much of their waking hours worrying about their own chances of death, as well as their children's chances, and their diaries and correspondence reflect this.

"As the time draws near I fear and tremble. I have suffered much in the last four weeks and often find myself indulging in forebodings of evil—of years of ill health as was the case before and all and the worst ills to be feared . . . God help me," wrote

Persis Sibley Andrews in her diary in 1847. A woman writes of her third birth in 1885, "Between oceans of pain there stretched continents of fear; fear of death and dread of suffering beyond bearing."*

Did male physicians bring intervention into childbirth?

Men brought intervention into childbirth as early as 1598 when Peter Chamberlen the Elder is credited with inventing the forceps. This development was kept secret by succeeding generations of Chamberlen family physicians until 1728. In the eighteenth century other physicians independently devised similar instruments, and forceps delivery came into widespread use.

The much-maligned cesarean section has been a human desire and practice from earliest times. Cesareans are mentioned in ancient Hindu, Egyptian, Grecian, Roman, and other folklore traditions. Of course it is assumed that the mother almost certainly did not survive the operation, which is one reason to believe that Caesar's surgical birth, despite Suetonius, was a legend. (His mother, Aurelia, apparently lived to hear of her son's invasion of Britain.) The first written record of both baby and mother surviving a cesarean comes from Switzerland in 1500 when Jacob Nufer performed the operation on his wife, after several days of unsuccessful labor and the ministrations of thirteen midwives. The mother lived to give birth to five more children, and the cesarean baby lived to be seventy-seven years old.

A woman conducted the first successful British cesarean section around 1815. James Miranda Stuart Barry performed the operation while masquerading as a man and serving as physician to the British

*Leavitt, *Brought to Bed.*

army in South Africa. As a quick little aside, nineteenth-century travelers in Africa also reported instances of indigenous people successfully carrying out the procedure with native medical practices. In 1879, R. W. Felkin witnessed a successful cesarean performed in Uganda. The healer used banana wine as a general anesthesia, sterilized both his hands and the woman's abdomen, used a midline incision, and applied cautery to minimize hemorrhaging. Afterward, the abdominal wound was pinned with iron needles and dressed with a root paste. The patient recovered, and Felkin concluded that the technique had been refined and in use for some time.*

Anesthesia during birth came on the American scene in 1847, when Fanny Appleton Longfellow became the first American woman to use ether during childbirth. Subsequently physicians used anesthetic agents, such as ether or chloroform or opium, in about half of physician attended births. In 1914, the "twilight sleep" procedure was imported from Germany. The now infamous twilight sleep was induced with a combination of scopolamine, a belladonna alkaloid and amnesiac, and morphine, an opiate. Women delivering with this method screamed and thrashed around even as their minds slept, and so were confined to a "crib-bed" to prevent injury. Women woke up from the experience feeling vigorous and remembering nothing. One of the foremost medical advocates of the procedure was a Dr. Bertha Van Hoosen. She called twilight sleep "the greatest boon the Twentieth Century could give women."†

---

*All references to cesarean section are taken from "Cesarean Section—A Brief History," prepared by Jane Eliot Sewell, Ph.D., for the American College of Obstetricians and Gynecologists in cooperation with the National Library of Medicine.

†Leavitt, *Brought to Bed.*

Did male physicians push female midwives out of the birthing process?

At the turn of the century, midwives still attended about half of the births in the United States. By the 1950s, the number of midwife-attended births dropped to 3 percent. The decline of midwives was due to the changing nature of health care economics and institutions, demographic changes, problems within the midwifery profession, and the desire of women to have physician-managed births and interventions. As Leavitt explains, middle- and upper-class women, as early as the mid-eighteenth century, saw physicians as a symbol of hope, as science's promise to end fear and suffering during childbirth and welcomed them and their interventions into their homes.

The depth of women's yearning to be freed from the rigors of childbirth, and their faith in science to deliver them, can be seen in the clamor for twilight sleep—in the face of opposition by a great number of male physicians. A National Twilight Sleep Association was formed, headed by active and prominent women's rights leaders, and including women doctors. Women saw the opportunity to be put to sleep and escape the pain of childbirth as an emancipating right, perceived the controversy as a fight for their sex, and pursued twilight sleep as a way of exerting control over the process of childbirth. Despite the fact that the *Journal of the American Medical Association* in 1914 declared that "this method has been thoroughly investigated, tried, and found wanting, because of the danger connected with it," women leaders were more afraid that the medical profession would keep them from its benefits. The movement suffered a setback in 1915 when Francis X. Carmody, one of the movement's foremost advocates, died during childbirth. After that, twilight sleep was limited to the first stage of labor. However, the technique and other narcotics were used routinely to alleviate pain and consciousness in childbirth through the 1960s.

Historically, did technological interventions lower mortality rates?

In many cases, interventions produced benefits, providing an increasing number of choices in childbirth for the mother and the physician. Forceps in the right hands could save the lives of both the mother and the child. Prior to forceps, a baby stuck in the birth canal could result in a double death. The only option, when changing positions or manual manipulation failed, would be to call a physician to perform a craniotomy on the baby with an instrument called the "crochet." Once the baby's brains were dissected and its cranium collapsed, the body could be removed from the mother.

Used inappropriately, however, the forceps could kill or maim both the mother and child. Further, once forceps became fashionable to use, they were overused, and often by physicians who were untrained and inexperienced. As Richard and Dorothy Wertz explain in *Lying-In: A History of Childbirth in America,** tools such as forceps, anesthesia, and ergot (a drug made from a naturally occurring fungus that could induce labor by causing powerful uterine contractions) once added to a physician's armamentarium, fed into the physician's need to "do something," as opposed to letting nature take its course.

When physicians were attending births in the home, the birth process was ultimately controlled by the mother and her attendants—midwives, friends, and relatives—who were female.

---

*Richard W. Wertz and Dorothy C. Wertz, *Lying-In: A History of Childbirth in America* (Yale University Press, 1989).

Under these circumstances, physicians often felt compelled to intervene to justify their existence, and their higher fees. Often, then, the intervention was unnecessary and dangerous, and actually added considerably to the mother and child's risk. This was a pattern that repeated itself with all the interventions that were introduced, foreshadowing the problems we have today. Technology at its best can bring more choices, added control, and more autonomy; at the same time, technology also brings costs that are seldom examined. Once used, a technological intervention—or let's call it innovation—is difficult to manage.

A far greater irony was that physicians killed far more women than they saved merely through their physical presence at the birth. Physicians carried infections to laboring women from their other patients. This was the famous "childbed fever" or puerperal infection,* which was the greatest killer of all. Even with the work of Ignaz Semmelweiss, a Viennese obstetrician who in 1861 advocated that physicians sanitize their hands and instruments, and Louis Pasteur's proof in 1879 that streptococcus was responsible for puerperal fever, physicians were unwilling to follow the new guidelines, lax in their implementation, and generally unable to prevent infection.

Judith Walzer Leavitt explains how the pattern of intervention and increased mortality reached its ultimate expression in the greatest intervention of all: the hospital. For women, the leap to hospitals came as a logical extension of their faith in science and the benefits that it promised. By the turn of the century, much of the reciprocal social network that made home births and traditional practices possible was gone. Hospitals represented a place

---

*Infection of the uterus and birth canal, usually caused by bacteria transmitted to the mother through the birth attendant's hands and instruments.

where women could go that was supposedly worry-free, consolidated all the benefits of science, and introduced a futuristic sense of convenience.

Obstetricians encouraged birth in hospitals as a way of finally achieving the sterile environment necessary to prevent puerperal infection, and as a way of consolidating their financial position and institutional power. OBs, as specialists, were looking to gain market share away from family practitioners and midwives, and their efforts mirrored the move toward specialization in the medical profession as a whole.

The move to the hospital environment also allowed obstetricians to experiment with early forms of actively managed birth. In 1920, Joseph B. DeLee, a leading light in the history of obstetrics, and a demon in the eyes of today's midwives and proponents of natural birth, declared birth to be a "pathologic process . . . and . . . only a small minority of women escape damage during labor. . . . So frequent are these bad effects, that I have often wondered whether Nature did not deliberately intend women to be used up in the process of reproduction, in a manner analogous to that of salmon, which dies after spawning?"

DeLee then devised an early version of the active management model. A typical DeLee birth would involve sedating the woman with scopolamine, waiting for cervical dilation, giving ether during the second stage of pregnancy, performing an episiotomy, and then using forceps to lift out the fetus. After the birth, he extracted the placenta, contracted the uterus with ergot, and closed the episiotomy incision. DeLee believed that this new procedure of his would save women's lives and make their postpartum periods less traumatic. Furthermore, the DeLee "prophylactic operation" represented a new move to make obstetrics scientific, systematic, and predictable by putting it in the hands of the specialist.

Things didn't work out the way DeLee or anyone imagined. Instead of reducing maternal mortality, the shift to hospitals actually increased it. The urban maternal mortality rate in the United States zoomed from forty-five per 10,000 at the turn of the century to well over seventy per 10,000 during the 1920s. The more women delivered in hospitals, the more they died.

To his credit, DeLee admitted the problem, blaming the "great evils, which swell the mortality and morbidity of the mothers and babies in the United States," on the practices of physicians and the structure of hospitals. Hospitals, by consolidating medical facilities, merely made it easier for infections to be carried from medical and surgical wards to obstetrical wards. Hospitals also made it easier to misuse interventions, because they, too, were more convenient.

The medical profession did manage to reform itself to a great degree, standardizing protocols and throttling back on the misuse of drugs and operative interventions. Admissions soared and hospital births rose from 35 percent of all births in 1933 to 72 percent by 1940, and hospitals lost their association with higher rates of puerperal deaths. By 1950 hospital births had risen to nearly 90 percent of all births, while midwife-attended births dropped to 3 percent. By 1960, hospital birth was nearly universal in the United States.

So what finally lowered maternal mortality rates from its high point of seventy-five per 10,000 births to its present rate of about one in 10,000? The answer to that question is not really obstetrics per se. As Leavitt points out, the discovery of penicillin in 1928 and its widespread use after World War II dramatically reduced mortality from postpartum infections, cesarean sections, and other complications, as it did in all medical disciplines. It was this ability to fight infection, combined with transfusions to replace blood lost to hemorrhaging, that finally conquered the two greatest killers of mothers and infants, and made childbirth a relatively safe event.

Are hospitals factories?

Hospitals eventually brought safety, but they also brought a pathological level of disassociation to birth and to the relationship between doctor and patient. American doctors lost touch with their patients, with the sense of the body, how the body lives out its life, and how the body is connected to a symbolic emotional life that humans hold dear. For this hubris, women have paid dearly.

The typical American birthing experience for most of the twentieth century is nothing to brag about. In the first third of the century, women moved from a risky but supportive familial setting to a risky, isolated, and impersonal arena. Even as mortality rates declined because of antibiotics, transfusions, and improved obstetrics protocols, doctors searched for ways of making safe births a more predictable and quantifiable commodity. The motivation? Not just the safety of the mother and child, but also the need for the efficiencies that lie at the heart of all modern institutions.

A laboring woman started out in what was euphemistically called a labor room. She was given painkillers, as well as scopolamine to remove the memory of pain. When she was ready to deliver, she was wheeled, in the middle of her contractions, to a "delivery" room, where she was placed on a table with stirrups. Her arms were strapped down and her legs were strapped high in the air. She lay in this strange position in a strange place in the middle of a thicket of equipment for anesthesia, transfusion, IV delivery, fetal heart monitoring, and neonatal resuscitation. She was given oxytocic drugs to counteract the effects of anesthesia and speed up the delivery. The routine use of forceps and the lithotomy position required routine episiotomy. And so on.

Most importantly, the woman faced this whole experience alone, cut off from her husband, family, friends, and other familiar supporters, and cut off from her own body. This disassociation has costs. One of the things you notice is that most women Julie's age have mothers and grandmothers who have absolutely no recollection of birth, and thus are unable to pass along any information of value—whether objective or emotional or ritual—to their daughters and granddaughters.

So, who's right?

As they say, only in America . . .

It's strange to take a step back from the OB-versus-midwife debate and try to get a little perspective. What's strange is to see all the inherent contradictions living side-by-side: our desire to have perfect babies next to our desire to have perfect experiences; the continuing expansion of birth-related technologies, and the desire for "natural" delivery. There are too many countervailing forces: It's just not going to work out the way people imagined.

American obstetricians have a lot to answer for. It is clear that many of the criticisms leveled at them today have been there from the very beginning—the distrust of bodily processes, the belief in intervention, the love of technology—and are justified. It's also important to realize that the criticism of American OBs comes from a great diversity of sources, not just midwives. The interventional nature of American birth has been criticized by the World Health Organization and by other disciplines within American medicine itself, most notably by family practitioners. In the future, American OBs will face increasing competition from other practitioners, arm-twisting from HMOs to contain their expensive habits, and increasing pressure from government agencies. Like AT&T, that other great monopoly which started at the beginning of the century, they're losing the franchise.

But you have to place the belief system of American OBs within a larger context. If American OBs are cultishly devoted to and reverential of technology, speed, and convenience, it is because they are the products of a culture whose creed is technology. Women were and are part of the historical forces that created the active management model of childbirth that exists today. When you think about it, it's a product that fulfills wishes that a majority of women held at the beginning of the century and still hold now: short, safe, convenient, and, if the patient desires, pain-free births. Midwives and feminist scholars who study childbirth fail to adequately understand and appreciate this.

Midwives deserve a lot of credit, and deserve to have their roles grow until they are major partners in the birthing industry. Studies indicate that they are more attentive; introduce earlier and better prenatal education and care; and produce equivalently safe, if not safer, results in the majority of cases they handle, with less intervention. If all goes well, they also have a much higher level of customer satisfaction.

But what midwives fail to understand is that what they do is also a system, a social process. There is no such thing as "natural" childbirth. Childbirth has the same relationship to nature that gardening has: It is a combination of nature and artifice, but certainly more artifice than nature. Everything we think of under the rubric of "health" is an integration of the biological and the social. Indeed, our bodies and how they work are to a large extent a function of what we eat, how clean our environment is, how often we receive medical attention, and what health practices and technologies we have at our disposal. All these things are a part of culture. All it takes to see this is to look at the differential in life span and reproductive mortality between first and third world nations.

So when midwives talk about natural birth, they are being somewhat disingenuous. Even in freestanding birthing centers, managed by midwives, an average of 15 to 20 percent of women are "risked-out" or referred to OB-managed programs. Another 15 to 20 percent on average are transferred to hospitals during labor and delivery for complications. Then another 2 to 5 percent of mothers and newborns are transferred postpartum for hospital care. So for roughly half of women, labor can safely proceed without technological intervention. For the other half, it's more complicated.

Which brings me to the problem of false expectations. If OBs do women a disservice by treating every delivery as a potential emergency, midwives provide a similar disservice by making women feel less than perfect if they need assistance. How "natural" can natural birth be if only half of women can achieve it? Not only do midwives inaccurately polarize the debate, they divide their own constituency. All around us, whether it's Julie's friends or conversations I overhear on the street, women feel somehow guilty if they had a C-section, or agreed to an episiotomy, or asked for pain relief (or, for that matter, felt pain at all). Instead, they should understand that birth is a continuum of contingencies that exists in a particular social environment.

The convenient fictions midwives peddle are ultimately paradoxical and self-defeating. When midwives would have you believe that women were brainwashed or forced into the present state of birth in America, they take away active moral and historical agency from women, and undermine their own position, and the position of all women. Why? Because most women understand all too well in their own hearts the fear their sisters felt a hundred years ago, the fear that drove the choices which were made, by both women and their doctors, and which sustain the system in place today. Perhaps this is a better, more honest, and more powerful place to start from than victimhood.

In the end there is also the problem of faith. At this point in time, I can hear what the midwives say, and much of it has the ring of truth. But when I look at Julie and her tummy and see the two most precious things in the world to me, I cannot put my faith in them. I cannot give up what I know. Not yet. For when I look at Julie's belly, I still see what the doctors see, what most of our culture sees. Not a simple natural process, not a Renaissance village with its walled garden, but a colossus of regulated mystery and complication, the domed city.

Here's something wild.

The spotted hyena gives birth through an extraordinary organ the size and shape of a penis. This birth method is so violent that often the penislike organ rips open. Or, just as often, the fetus gets stuck within the tube. Researchers estimate that 65 to 70 percent of firstborn young and 18 percent of first-time mothers die.

Squirrel monkeys have such a tight fit between birth canal and fetal head and body size that labor obstruction is common: Sixteen percent of squirrel monkeys are stillborn, and 34 percent die of birth-related injuries soon after birth.

See Julie, it could be a lot worse.

Humans aren't the only animals in nature who have a hard time giving birth. This morning over breakfast Julie and I are checking out another anthropological and zoological wonkfest in the *Times* science section—"Why Babies Are Born Facing Backward, Helpless, and Chubby."

The hyena's strange birth organ and high birth mortality can be accounted for by high levels of androgens, or male hormones, that bathe hyenas while they are in the womb. The baby hyenas who make it come out jaws snapping, ready to rock 'n' roll. Similarly, certain species of monkeys need fully developed brains at birth so they can immediately swing through the 3-D world of a rainforest canopy and feed themselves.

Nature makes compromises on birth to achieve certain advantages. The compromise nature made with humans came with encephalization, or the development of large brain size. While most of the human brain's development comes after birth, the brain and the cranium are still large enough to present a tight fit through the pelvic opening—no doubt a piece of evolutionary engineering that resulted in a great deal of maternal and infant mortality.

The most fascinating theory of human birth comes from Wenda Trevathan, a specialist in evolutionary medicine from New Mexico State University. Her ideas suggest how strong an influence human emotions and emotional support have in the birth process, and how important birth-connected emotions were in human evolution.

First, changes in the shape of the human pelvis during transition to bipedalism resulted in the need for assistance during the birthing process. In quadrupedal primates, the baby descends straight through the birth canal and arrives at the vaginal outlet face up. This allows the mother to assist the baby, such as by pulling the baby out, or unwinding an umbilical cord from the baby's neck, or clearing the nose and airway of mucus so the baby can start breathing-procedures that can mean the difference between life and death.

The evolution of bipedalism canceled all these benefits and increased the risks of mortality. The birth canal was reoriented so that the widest spans of the pelvic opening and the vaginal outlet are perpendicular to each other. The baby has to execute a series of rotations through the birth canal to pass the widest part of the head as well as the shoulders. The end result, and the critical issue to Trevathan's hypothesis, is that the baby arrives at the birth outlet facing away from the mother. Because of the awkwardness of this delivery presentation, the mother cannot reach the neck or the airway, or if she tries to pull the baby out, she risks spinal damage.

The transition from the individual to the social nature of childbirth may date back as far as the ancestral females of the Miocene epoch (5 million years ago)—before hominids and before language. Trevathan hypothesizes that these females probably decided where to deliver their infants, what position to be in for delivery, and perhaps even when to deliver. Three million years later, as encephalization increased and our ancestors evolved into humans, females became conscious of their vulnerability during childbirth and began seeking out others for emotional as well as physical support during delivery. Females who felt a great deal of anxiety in anticipation of birth and sought assistance at the time of delivery had more surviving offspring than those who continued the ancient mammalian pattern of delivering alone.

The emotions that surround childbirth, such as fear, anxiety, doubt, and uncertainty, are human adaptations to the birthing complications resulting from bipedalism, and in turn led to the social relationships, the joint communication, and the cooperative behavior among women that we recognize today in the midwifery model. It also can be seen as the first obstetrical intervention, and the beginning of the transfer of authority for birth out of the hands of the individual mother and into the hands of her attendants.

Trevathan takes the role of emotions in labor one step further by suggesting that emotional and social support go beyond just positive feelings about birth to actually having an effect on the success of the birth process itself. Not only do women naturally seek out emotional support at birth, that emotional support—as recent studies have conclusively shown—has a profoundly positive biomechanical effect, resulting in easier births, reduced pain, and fewer complications.

What's interesting to me about Trevathan's ideas is the way they embody all the issues we're still going through today. The profound fear associated with childbirth, the need for birth attendants, the surrendering of individual authority to a social system, the biomechanical effect of emotional support, the impact of environment, the tension between autonomy and trust—they are all part of our biological origins.

There's no question in my mind that the evolution of a culture of childbirth had enormous benefits to our ancestors. Heightened emotionality, social contact and cooperation, rituals, and ultimately language are adaptive responses and tools that our ancestral women used to bring some order to creation. Their attempts to make sense of birth created a lineage of instruction, a cooperative legend, a tool to mediate some of their greatest fears. What more heroic example of wits than using language as a tool to deal with a nature relentlessly intent on random experimentation?

This is a concept even a man can understand.

What greater example of the ongoing dialog between nature and culture operating simultaneously within our own bodies than the example of women today mobilizing to take back the story of birth? Doesn't someone hear an ancestral echo?

• • •

"Even before I was pregnant, I knew how I wanted to do it. I always saw myself as having lots of children, as moving around a lot during labor, making a lot of noise. That's how I express myself in my dance and in other ways."

Since our own pregnancy worries had brought her to mind, it seemed only appropriate that we call and catch up with our friend Willow. So much of what she went through in that cabin in the Vermont woods perfectly captured our ambivalence and our fears. After Julie chatted with her a while, I got on the line and asked her to tell me the story of her labor and delivery.

"I lined myself up with a midwife who looked at everything as a natural process. The whole experience of going to the midwife for my prenatal was so nice and affirming. The pregnancy went along with no particular warning signs in the meantime. So we thought we could continue with that attitude and that everything would be fine—the baby would just flow.

"It was in December, and labor started gradually. There was a snowstorm, and I was told to keep walking, so I did all sorts of things to try to make the labor come on stronger, because it wouldn't come. It would sort of fade, and then it would come again. We were all sort of waiting for it to really kick in.

"I took walks out in the snow. I'd lean against a tree, and watch the flakes fall. I'd have my neighbor massage my back. I didn't want to lie down at all. We sang a lot. The only time where I really felt that I could let go of my helpers was when I was in the bath. I didn't feel the pain so much in the bathtub.

"The first stage of labor went on for about thirty-six hours. The labor would just stall out every night, around two. I never got to transition point or pushing. The baby wasn't pushing down enough to open up the cervix, so my contractions weren't efficient. That's what they said.

"Somehow, this thing that I never thought could happen was happening. It was out of my control, my body was failing me. I wasn't going to make happen by doing all the right things and drinking all the right herbs, and being physical, and having all the right images. This was shocking to me.

"On the third night, I gave up. Stephen was really overwhelmed by having to watch me in so much pain. By then we both knew it wasn't happening. He was crying and I was crying, and we said, okay, it's time for somebody else to do something for us.

"The moment I walked into the hospital I was 'tsked at' for coming in so late. It was like 'Okay, bring 'em in. You tried to do this crazy thing, and we got the baby anyway in the end.' 'Failed home birth' is what they called it. I had my water broken. I was hooked up with an IV. I was prepped for surgery. It was just a really different feeling. You just become a patient.

"In the end I was just so relieved that I could rest now, and that in half an hour I could see the baby. The spinal was a wonderful thing, too. I stayed awake. They just gave me a shot that got rid of my lower half. I had been in back labor, and it had been a grinding kind of nerve-twisting thing, so I was glad when it went away.

"Birth is the most dramatic single thing that happens to an adult woman. It has a great potential for making you feel empowered. I feel envy when I hear women who have had vaginal birth tell their war stories. They like to talk about how painful it was and how they overcame it. It wasn't until my second pregnancy and my second C-section that I really understood the impact on me. I had had so many strong and vivid images of giving birth, and it never happened. It had been such a deep assumption about my life.

"It's very hard to feel the triumph of owning a birth when someone else cuts your baby out for you. You have to surrender. You have to be put out. You have to be cut. You feel miserable the first twenty-four hours of your baby's life. You can't stand up. You can't really nurse. You're feeling bliss, but you're in agony. That's not powerful.

"The doctors told me, other women told me, 'You have a healthy baby, what's the difference?' There's a lot of significance about how you come into the world. For nine months you have so much control. You're controlling how the baby's fed, what the baby hears. Suddenly, in the end to have everything taken away from you—it's a really big loss. Birth is the last moment when you can really feel that you are creating this person's life, and I couldn't.

"True, if I had lived in another time, I would have been dead. I wouldn't have had a baby. The second time I tried just about everything I could think of, but nature didn't come. Things just weren't right. That's the mystery."

MONTH SIX

FEAR, SEX, AND LOATHING

To those who say men's brains are in their penises, I say
thinking of any kind, even at the pelvic level, is not con-
ducive to sex.

Actually today I am able to report that I am finally a happy
man. After a month-long batting slump I have finally been able to
perform my conjugal duties. I know it sounds strange—a married
man feeling ambivalent about making love to his wife—or perhaps
not so strange. Whatever the case, I have to admit it has not been
easy for me lately. It seems that Mr. Weenie has achieved a certain
level of self-consciousness and that is not a good thing. While the
party line is that Julie remains "my beautiful partner to whom I am
devoted," to Mr. Weenie, she is beginning to look like a cross
between Danny DeVito in *Batman Returns* and the Bubble Girl in
Hieronymous Bosch's *Gates of Hell*.

In the very beginning, right after we found out Julie was pregnant, sex was actually more fun. It felt like we were reenacting
some important event in history. The Conception: Take #2. Also,
lost was that feeling that started in teenager-hood with all that

fumbling around in parking lots and the backrooms of parties, of sex being only about self-gratification. Replaced by something else: a sense that you had pushed open the doors of the pulsating Disco of Orgasm, and stepped into the clear refreshing night of a future. The mutuality of it felt positive, as well as a little bit kinky.

But soon other feelings crept in. The onset of nausea didn't do wonders for Julie's libido, and it made me feel, if I was "in the mood," that I was trying to push myself on a sick person. Plus, it usually took only one look at the bedside box of crackers, and the waiting plastic garbage pail, to turn my thoughts to onanism.

By the third month Julie's nausea had passed and her libido had returned with a vengeance. That was when I began to notice. For instead of returning her ardor, I felt tentative, and avoided her and our bed with a reticence bordering on virginal. Finally, one night as I looked down at her—postcoitally—it occurred to me what it was. Her middle was thickening. This was not the cute thorax I had married.

From there it got worse, trust me.

First, I have to give myself a break. Somehow curling up together and sharing Julie's favorite bedtime reading, *The Birth Partner*, did not work out brilliantly as foreplay. But as long as Julie more or less looked the same, things held together.

In month five when Julie's belly suddenly popped from her midsection like bubblegum from a teenager's lips, things really started falling apart. I mean it's one thing to look across the street at a pregnant woman gliding along dressed in a flowing shift and say something like: "Oh, isn't creation sensuous." It's quite another thing to lie in bed staring at a beachball of flesh with veins running through it.

Now that the baby is moving, Julie has developed this unsettling habit of continually stroking her stomach no matter where she is. It goes something like this: stroke . . . stroke . . . stroke . . . pat . . . pat . . . pat . . . "Ooh, Gordon, did you see that? She moved!" Followed by a little squeal of joy. All I can say is that it was wondrous the first time and fun the next fifty times, but by now I'm beginning to feel like the spectator who couldn't find the exit at Sea World.

It's bad enough when we're in supermarkets where innocent bystanders are trying to buy food, or in restaurants where other people are trying to eat, but at least in those venues I can distract myself. In bed, there is no escape. Picture me with my head desperately buried in some magazine. I get a tap on the arm. I look over to see the flesh on Julie's belly deflecting and rippling wildly as the little passenger kicks out against the wall of her compartment. I smile wanly and nod my head in mutuality, but all I can think about is that scene in *Alien*. Then Julie looks at me with a mantis gleam in her eye.

One night in the middle of lovemaking—which is touchy now at best, because I'm beginning to feel like Julie and I are connected by an aquarium—I feel the baby *kick me* through Julie's stomach. Let us just say it had an effect on me akin to O-ring failure on the space shuttle.

And then there are the nightmares . . . like the one where I hear droning and look up to see Julie's belly looming over Lakehurst, New Jersey.

Oh, the humanity.

The world is divided neatly into two camps: couples who enjoy sex during pregnancy and couples who don't.

A quick poll among my male friends reveals that I am not the only squeamish one. My friend William reports decorously that the "urge for sex just went away." Also, as he was "doing it" he kept wondering if he would "hurt the baby." He kept imagining that he would touch the baby with the head of his penis, and he felt "it was the wrong place to put the thing."

Fear of hurting the baby is a common theme among the "just say no to pregnancy sex" crowd. There is also the problem of adjusting to changes in your partner's body—kind of a "this isn't what I signed up for" response. Joseph starts out by trying to describe it as a "series of mechanical problems," and ends up with "like trying to make love to a whale." Gary talks about the "tummy being too large for good contact," and "smells and gas not being particularly sexy," as well as "things being big and loose all around."

Then there are the examples of how you handle your pregnant partner's feelings and insecurities about her changing body. My friend Robbie, always a good representative for the sensitive fin-de-siècle male, recalls telling his wife, Darien, she was "a hard-boiled egg on stilts," a relatively subtle metaphor compared to when he simply called her "a big fat cow." "I guess I was pretty rough on her," Robbie mused. "Partly it was my clumsy attempt to introduce a little humor into the situation. The other part was me wanting to give her grief." Atta boy, Robbie. No latent hostility there.

On top of the physical changes are the psychological ones. There is the incest angle, the hint of taboo I felt lurking in the bed. Adam, the professional Oedipist, weighs in with a blunt, "I was never into being aroused by a mother." Sniffing, he continues, "Some men are into it, sucking the milk and everything." William worried that Claire "was going to turn into her sister, who is a very mothering and very nurturing person." And back to Robbie: "I married this beautiful blond woman who was fun to be with and fun in bed. One day I turn around and it's like I married my mother. Which is when I realized that I actually hate my mother."

Isn't it ironic? What gives so much pleasure one moment, six months later is either repulsive or done out of a sense of obligation. I imagine for men who are "with it," making love to your pregnant wife is not so much about lust and self-gratification as it is about giving support and encouragement, and signaling commitment during a period when a woman is feeling vulnerable about her looks, her ability to attract. That is why in quieter, less selfish moments, I have regrets. Julie has never seemed happier. I surprise myself when I realize that I've actually stopped worrying about her unassisted mental state. But it's more than that. While Julie's body thickens, her spirit is growing loose-limbed and light. Despite her increasing bulk, she is as graceful in her bliss—moving about, doing her work, and making her preparations deftly and purposefully as Wayne Gretzky skating down the ice with the puck.

I feel bad that I cannot share these feelings. Sex would be the right gesture at this point. The mutual physicality of it would be a gift, a way of sharing Julie's present joie de vivre as well as a way to reassure Julie that she is still attractive to me, and that our bonds still hold.

I have even gone so far as to consult sex manuals while skulking in the remote sections of finer bookstores to see what advice they might offer. Alas, most of them recommend doing it in a dark, weightless environment.

But nothing is more confounding to me as when I consult the other half of the world—my friends who actually enjoyed sex during pregnancy. Howard, a composer, claimed that the whole situation was extremely romantic for him. "For me the pregnancy was symbolic of our love for each other, and so it seemed logical to continue making love. I liked all of the physical changes. The swelling of her belly and her breasts were lovely— not necessarily erotic, but lovely. There was always the issue of being careful and restrained, but that was not necessarily a negative. I remember our lovemaking as sweet and gentle."

Stephen also enjoyed the physical changes. "I wasn't upset by the physical changes. Just the opposite, I got a more bodacious version of Maggie! Plus, sex in general was more exciting and carefree. We didn't have to use birth control. Also, at times, I felt so removed from the pregnancy that sex was a way for me to get close and share in the experience. I also have to admit that it was a way for me to get some attention during this new thing that was changing our lives."

No one was more passionate about his sex life during pregnancy (and pregnancy in general) than Jesse. I was over at his apartment in Park Slope having a cup of coffee, bemoaning the flaming wreckage of my sex life. Dorothy, his slim, blond wife, was darting around in the background, taking care of their two-year old, Ian—a nice counterpoint to Jesse, who is a bearlike mensch.

"For all boys, pregnancy can be construed as a betrayal. All of a sudden the boy who has the sole attention and sexual favor of the woman in his life, finally, is now being betrayed by the fetus and her body, and by the fact that he's not a boy anymore and he has to be responsible."

Does that mean you had a hard time with sex during Dorothy's pregnancy?

No. I really loved my wife's body when she got pregnant. I LOVED IT. My wife is skinny and is not ample chested . . . So I thought that this complete transformation from a petite woman to this beautiful, voluptuous mother-to-be was just so wonderful. For me pregnant women are really sexy. I like that kind of Mother Nature image. I took a lot of pictures of her pregnant— just of her belly—as well as some nudes of her pregnant.

So what you're telling me is that feeling positive about pregnancy is all about the transformation from an A to a C cup?

No. The sexual aspect of the pregnancy was just one part of it. The whole experience was a glorious time for the both of us. I don't think anyone's sexual relationship after eight years of marriage is perfect. It is what it is. And every relationship has aspects that are wonderful as well as destructive, and you bring all of that into sex. So certainly that was there, but to a lesser extent because of the excitement of the pregnancy. And we were literally excited for nine months.

What do you think made it a different experience for you than for so many other guys?

Maybe it was because I could see my new family literally in the making. Maybe it's because I am also very inquisitive and curious about change. I wanted to be as much a part of the pregnancy and birth as possible. I always used to say that if could put a breast on, I would help feed. I was so fascinated by the whole process all the way through, through the episiotomy which she had to have because she was tearing. I wanted to see how it was done. That's who I am though. It was a new adventure and discovery. And some people don't look at it this way.

Didn't you have any hard times?

Yeah, but in a way, it helped with the bond between Dorothy and me. My wife had gestational diabetes, which meant that she had to be very careful about her diet, and take blood four times a day. The dietary thing became a game or a process. She had to lance her finger and take a glucose level, which is unpleasant. We recorded it in a book, and I carried the book. Whatever we did it became a little process, a little ritual, a little regimen. It became part of my overall responsibility in the pregnancy, which was to make sure the nest was comfortable and to make sure she felt safe and secure and loved.

It seems like you guys really synched up with each other, really figured out how to communicate and cooperate? How can this be?

I will never take credit for the pregnancy. By the same token, I will say that my wife was good enough to let me share as much I could handle and wanted, and as much capacity as I could take, and wanted to share with me as much as she could.

The value of cooperation is something I understand from my work. I'm a cameraman. I like cooperation and collaboration. When I'm on the job, we're all working together to make a movie or to make a TV show. If someone doesn't do his job, then the whole thing fails. If everyone pulls together, you create a pretty glorious production, which is very fulfilling. That's what I wanted to bring to the pregnancy. A real sharing of experience.

It all sounds very symbolic. What do you think it revealed in you?

The need for family and the realization that I was going to have family really revealed to me my adulthood. When Dorothy became pregnant, it all clicked.

It brought together things that started happening for me when my mother died. When I was twenty-nine my mother came to me and said, "I've had a relapse of the cancer I had ten years ago." I knew at that point this was going to be terminal. She said, "I want to go home and I'd like it if you could take care of me." There was animosity between me and my mother. But I turned around and I said, "I'm there for you, whatever happens we'll get through it." So for six months I stopped working. I was there for her. I took the mantle and felt very proud and very fulfilled by it. And when she died, I knew that I had done something and that I had completed a certain thing. Going out into the world after I buried my mom, I knew that I was capable. My mother's death was a very liberating process. I was ready to become an adult.

When I realized that my wife was pregnant, I said to myself, Let's see if I can take things one step further. Let me see if I am an adult who can be a kind, loving, caring father. I separated the wheat in my life from the chaff. I got down to fundamentals. I realized I had a responsibility to both my child and to my wife to make the experience as positive as possible for the both of them. So, when the baby came into the world, he was coming into an environment of love and support rather than one of jealousy, animosity, or misgiving in any form. You realize that the material things you have are secondary to "Are you loved? Do you love? Do you have a family that will be by your side?"

The idea of fatherhood was the idea of potential for me instead of fear, which I think it can be for a lot of men. They say, "Don't! Wait until you're ready!" I was actually ready. I was aching to have a child. I feel that in the wisdom of the deaths I have lived through, I have grown to understand that there is more value to life than to things. And that part of the adventure for me is the responsibility and the risk I'm choosing to take.

•   •   •

After slinking home from my talk with Jesse, all I could think about was, "All that from a question about sex?"

Later that night, after Julie was safely asleep, I forced myself to look at her belly. For the first time I reached out to touch it, unbidden. I stroked it gently to the rhythm of her soft snoring.

All that our pregnancy revealed in me is how confused I am. How ambivalent I am about responsibility. How much of my life had been built around, if not outright avoiding responsibility, at least diminishing its drag on my daily life.

I was also haunted by Jesse's use of the word "adventure." It is a word every boy loves. And yet, why could I not relate to our experience with such a word?

Looking down at the veins in her belly before slipping into sleep, I have the sensation of looking down from a great height at one of the great primitive rivers of the world, the Congo, or the Amazon. It is a metaphor I cannot resist. Life-giving, essential, impenetrably mysterious.

The Huaorani of the Amazon would have happily accepted Jesse Nadelman into their tribe. He would have made a great Huaorani husband. The similarities are amazing.

I'm not joking. I'm back in the library reading about couvade, or more specifically the Huaorani couvade, in a paper by Laura Rival, an anthropologist from the University of Kent.* A Huaorani man "will stop eating fish and most types of meat.... Starting from the time the woman enters labor until a few days after the birth of the child, the husband restricts his food intake to boiled plantain

---

*Laura Rival, "Androgynous Parents and Guest Children: Huaorani Couvade," *Journal of the Royal Anthropological Institute*, December 1998.

or manioc broth. He avoids hunting and stays at home as much as possible . . ."

The specific foods and circumstances were different, but I can't help thinking about Jesse helping Dorothy follow her diabetic diet and the importance he attached to it. What bears the greatest similarity to Jesse and Dorothy's pregnancy is that couvade to the Huaorani is not a male rite, but a *couple rite.* Both parents are anxious to protect the fetus, and both parents share equally in the creation of the child.

There are plenty of other similarities. Just as Jesse mentioned that pregnancy revealed his adulthood to him, for the Huaorani couple, having a child is a sign of the passage into adulthood for both of the parents. Adulthood is about pairing up and having children, creating new social beings, adding to the community. Indeed, couvade for the Huaorani acts as a second marriage, a mutual rite of passage. The birth of a child makes an enduring couple out of the parents, and the husband and wife are reborn as father and mother during the birth process.

There's more. Just as Jesse got involved throughout the pregnancy and childbirth process itself, "Huaorani men do not 'imitate' childbirth, but take an active part in it, often acting as midwives. . . . The expectant father helps his wife during labor by massaging her back. He applies stinging nettles—a common analgesic—on her stomach, back, and temples. He may reach into his wife's body if there is a difficulty, as when, for instance, the umbilical cord is wrapped around the baby's neck. He also knows how to assist her in breech deliveries. The father cuts the umbilical cord with a knife-shaped piece of bamboo, wraps the placenta in the large leaves on which the baby was born, and buries the bundle with the afterbirth in the nearby forest. His mother-in-law may aid a young husband in all these tasks, until he acquires sufficient knowledge and experience. He might do no more than observe her during the birth of his first child. But by the third or fourth delivery, the roles are reversed; the prospective father is in charge."

The convergence is amazing. Both Jesse and the Huaorani believe that parental and social bonding begin before birth. Both use ritual to actualize these ideas, and both incorporate and integrate the pregnancy experience as a fundamental, "activating" metaphor in the story of their life.

Amazing. A whole tribe of Jesse Nadelmans. Someone alert the American Anthropological Association.

What have we really learned, what do we really know about fathers and their lives?

If you glance at the psychological literature of the last fifty years, as I'm doing, you might wonder. Most of the ideas belong in a boneyard. It's like walking through a museum of natural history, you know, the ones with dinosaur skeletons.

As I read through all this stuff the one word that comes to mind concerning the role of expectant fathers is "plight." If midwives criticize OBs for treating pregnant women as if they were physically ill, one could accuse the psychiatric establishment of doing the same thing to expectant men, the illness associated with pregnancy in this case being mental. Some of the titles are truly startling, like "The Psychosis of Fatherhood," "Psychosis in Males Relating to Fatherhood," "Fatherhood as a Precipitant of Mental Illness," and the ever popular "Sexually Deviant Behavior in Expectant Fathers."

If you don't have categories to deal with something, you see past it. If you have the wrong categories, you distort it. It makes me wonder whether the puzzle of "seeing" and understanding our own behavior as "modern" people is caused by the sciences and not resolved by them—caused by their inability to ask the right questions, use the right metaphors, tell the right tales? Is life really so much more complicated than Jesse or the Huaorani explain it? Or do we have to settle for timorous explanations such as: "while no specific criteria have been developed to establish that expectant fatherhood constitutes a universal developmental phase or sub-phase, it has been commonly accepted that parenthood represents a developmental process."

The point here is that for thousands and maybe tens of thousands and maybe hundreds of thousands of years societies have been treating expectant fatherhood as a distinct phase, a time of profound symbolic importance as well as pronounced anxieties, as evidenced by the rituals that structure and explain it. Psychology, however, hasn't quite gotten to this point.

Becoming a Father: A Psychoanalytical Perspective on the Forgotten Parent, by Michael Diamond, supports this view. He starts out by saying that psychology and the social sciences have neglected the father in the early stages of parenting, describes the father as the "forgotten parent" in the psychoanalytic literature, and suggests that neglect by the sciences has contributed to the devaluation of the father's role.

Diamond also points out succinctly one of the major problems that men have concerning their role as parents: "the parental ambitions of the boy and man, their urges to create life, have generally remained linked to the maternal, woman ambitions and prerogatives. . . . It is almost, one senses, as if to be a parent one must be a woman."

He notes that some "husbands . . . feel . . . excluded from their wives and the 'creature within her,' who may come to be viewed as a rival." He catalogs the differing dynamics that some men have with sex during pregnancy, reporting "changes in the male's psychosexual responses when confronted by the more dramatic changes in his wife's physical appearance." Finally, he mentions something that it totally curious. "Many fathers become concerned with gastrointestinal and other somatic symptoms, including couvade. . . . Issues from this phase are followed by hermaphroditic fantasies wherein the boy sees himself as able to both fertilize and bear children—able to carry a baby like a mother while sustaining himself within the male role. This is manifest in the expectant father in the wish to 'have it both ways.'"

This I can relate to. I certainly have had fantasies about bringing up our child alone. Jesse certainly had them. The Huaorani created a whole myth based around it.

Deep down inside, maybe we all have a little sea horse in us?

That word again, "couvade." Except this time it appears to mean something different.

During computer searches, I have been noticing medical and nursing journal citations with the word "couvade" in the title, mixed in with the usual anthropological articles. The first time it happened I ignored it, but as I scan down my search results, the numbers of these articles are building. Finally, I go in for a closer look.

The temperature in the General Reading Room of the New York Public Library must be close to ninety degrees. After pulling up several articles and quickly reading the abstracts, my vision starts to narrow, and I feel a slight sense of chill.

"The majority of expectant fathers in this study (87%) reported one or more symptoms during pregnancy, with at least 70% of the sample reporting one or more symptoms in each stage of pregnancy."*

*O. L. Strickland, "The Occurrence of Symptoms in Expectant Fathers," *Nursing Research*, 1986.

"Over the 11 months of their participation in the study, the vast majority of expectant fathers (93.7% to 97%) reported they experienced at least one *couvade* symptom in a typical month."*

"In a general medical practice, staffed by general internists and nurse practitioners, 22.5% of men with pregnant wives sought care for symptoms related to pregnancy that could not be otherwise objectively explained. . . ."†

Apart from what we know as ritual couvade, reported by anthropologists and travelers, men with actual physiological pregnancy symptoms are a part of common folklore. Until the 1960s, men who reported these symptoms were treated, as one paper put it, as a "neurotic minority." Then, in 1965, Sir William H. Trethowan, one of Britain's foremost psychiatrists, conducted a study into what he called the "couvade syndrome." He found that, despite the absence of any apparent disease, expectant fathers reported a variety of symptoms that mimic the symptoms of pregnant women. These include indigestion, abdominal pain, food cravings, nausea and vomiting, increased or decreased appetite, weight gain, constipation, headache, toothache, nosebleed, itch, muscle tremors, rashes, extreme fatigue, and an assortment of other aches and pains. The incidence of the symptoms appeared over the duration of the pregnancy in a U-shaped curve, with an increase in the first trimester, a decrease in the second, and another increase in the third. Trethowan conducted several studies. In one, he reported that one in nine of the expectant fathers he studied had couvade syndrome. In another, the rate was much higher, 50 percent.

*"Expectant Fathers at Risk for Couvade," *Nursing Research*, 1986.
†M. Lipkin and G. S. Lamb, "The Couvade Syndrome: An Epidemiological Study," *Annals of Internal Medicine*, 1982.

Since Trethowan's work, numerous other researchers, mostly in Western industrialized nations, conducted similar studies with remarkable results. Studies in the United States in Boston, Baltimore, Rochester, and Milwaukee found an incidence rate for couvade syndrome that ranged from 22.5 percent to over 90 percent. A Swedish study recorded 20 percent. A recent (1993) study in Thailand reported a 61 percent incidence in Thai men.

The discrepancies can be explained by the differing methodologies used and the differing definitions of couvade syndrome-whether, for example, nonphysical symptoms or particular mental states, such as bouts of irritability or sleeplessness, would be counted. Also, another difficulty is the high background prevalence of these symptoms. In other words, people have plenty of backaches, headaches, stomachaches, etc., without expecting or being pregnant. Studies have different methods for controlling for these symptoms, or differentiating between pregnancy-related and non-pregnancy-related symptoms.

Even the most conservative and cautious American study, conducted by a physician, Lipkin, and a nurse-practitioner, Lamb, in Rochester, New York, reported a high incidence of couvade syndrome, 22.5 percent. The actual rate could have been much higher, since they examineed the health care-seeking rate of expectant men, counting expectant fathers who actually went so far as to consult a physician for their symptoms. Second, they had a very conservative definition of couvade symptoms, focusing on a narrow range of physical symptoms: nausea and vomiting; abdominal pain or bloating; changes in appetite, weight, or bowel movements; elusive toothaches; concern about skin lesions, or growths, or cysts; leg cramps; faintness and lassitude or extreme fatigue. Other pregnancylike symptoms, such as ankle swelling and water retention, genital burning and itching, groin pain, and knee and upper leg pain, were *noted* but not included. Psychological states and changes were also not included. Third, they had two control periods. If a man had similar symptoms in either the six-month period leading up to the pregnancy or six months after, he was excluded, even though his specific symptoms during the pregnancy period could have been couvade-related.

Even with all these restrictions, Lipkin and Lamb reported nearly one in four men with couvade syndrome in their article in the April 1982 edition of the *Annals of Internal Medicine*. They concluded their report with: "The choice of symptoms was intentionally conservative. Qualitative review of these cases showed that many other symptoms may have had this cause. . . . These sorts of considerations lead us to conclude that our design underestimates the prevalence of couvade syndrome."

Some studies speculated as to why the body exhibits or "somatizes" physical symptoms. Frankly, no one has a good explanation for somatization. Most scientific and laymen's guesses rely on the idea that the body symptomizes certain psychological states, such as anxiety. Trethowan speculated that the syndrome occurs in societies where the ritual couvade is not practiced, thus linking the two through a sort of inverse logic. One study suggested that it is a means by which men can participate more fully in the birth cycle. Another speculates that couvade syndrome may be an expression of profound caring for the partner and unborn child. Yet another links ritual couvade with couvade syndrome by saying that both represent normal responses to a developmental crisis.

After several hours of reviewing this material I was left with an odd combination of exhilaration, numbness, and doubt. The explanations for the couvade syndrome were what gave me the most pause. The idea that psychological states can cause physical symptoms is a long-held view in the psychiatric and medical sciences, but the ideas floated by most of these studies seemed fanciful. What was obvious was that nobody had the faintest idea why it happened, the main reason I assume that this body of research isn't more widely known.

Despite the wide variation in the data, however, I felt sure that couvade syndrome, or physiological couvade, actually existed. In fact, Lipkin and Lamb's study, which came in with the lowest numbers, seemed to me to be the best proof. If one in four was the result of an extremely conservative study, what were the possibilities for the actual figures? A quick thought flitted through my brain. What if the methodologies used by researchers were too crude to capture all the symptoms in expectant men? What if the actual prevalence of couvade syndrome was nearly 100 percent?

Under the great dome of the General Reading Room, I took a few minutes to download and print out some articles I didn't have time to read. I had that feeling, the feeling that something you thought was peripheral, even slightly ridiculous, is actually the center of the universe. The type of sensation I'm sure that the former high school classmates of Bill Gates now feel.

"I was very interested in the general phenomenon that occurs in medicine of people experiencing physical symptoms for which there's no physiological or anatomical explanation."

I had called Mack Lipkin on a lark, picking his number off the title page of his study in the *Annals of Internal Medicine*. He was the coauthor, along with Gerri S. Lamb, of "The Couvade Syndrome: An Epidemiological Study." His office at Bellevue Hospital was a warren of books, piled on the floor, on chairs and desks, falling out of overstuffed bookshelves. This was the office of a working scientist.

"The easiest way is to think about it as a transduction of a

psychosocial experience into physical experience. It may work the same way *synesthesia* works."

Huh?

It's a condition in which one type of stimulation evokes the sensation of another, like when a certain sound produces the visualization of a color. The "blues" in music, for example.

The way sonar works? A transducer takes waves that travel through water and turns them into electromagnetic readings?

Yeah, exactly. A transducer is a device that accepts an input of energy in one form and produces an output of energy in some other form. This is essentially what happens in the body. For example, it can be very positive. When you're in love, you get a warm feeling. Sometimes it's very negative, like: "You're a pain in the ass." If you listen to the language, it may just sound like a semantic thing, but people feel these things in their bodies. If you don't believe me, go to a scary movie.

Anyway, as I was saying, I was looking for the right situation to study people who had somatic symptoms when I got lucky. As Pasteur said, "Chance favors the prepared mind." An acquaintance, who is also a patient of mine, walks into my office one day. I had treated him perhaps twenty-five times over the last seven years. He had always had a skin tag on his neck, a sort of big wart about the size of the end of a pinky, which would pop out from under his collar. I would always offer to take it off for him, as it occasionally got red and irritated, and it was the type of thing people would stare at in meetings, but he would always wave me off and say, "It's fine, it's fine." So one day he comes in very agitated and says, "I've

got to have this thing off right away." I asked him why. "Because it's driving me crazy, I can't stand it." I said, "It looks the same to me, has something changed?" He said, "No, I'm just sick of it and it's driving me nuts. I just want it off. Can you take it off right now?"

So, I took it off. He thanked me and as he turned to leave he said, "Oh, by the way, my wife's pregnant." And he left. Well, they were both my patients. I knew they weren't looking to have another child. They had two children, one of whom was a Down's syndrome child. This new pregnancy was six years after their last child, and I knew it was unintended. I thought about it and it rang a bell for me, that this was a sudden anxious concern about a new growth. I started looking for it in the medical literature, and this seemed a very good example of couvade syndrome.

Coincidentally, I was attending on the wards at the same time. The house staff presented a case to me, a guy with abdominal pain, saying, "This guy's very sick and we don't know what's wrong with him. He's got nausea and vomiting, abdominal swelling and pain." He was a young construction worker, street tough with tattoos and a macho style. He had been in a lot of fights, he had scarring on his face. The residents are telling me they've tried X-rays, and now they want to do a blind aspiration of his abdomen—basically, stick a needle in their and see what they could find. This was in the days before MRI and laparoscopy. So I'm sitting there listening, and all of a sudden it struck me that this sounds like pregnancy! So I said, "Let me talk to him a little bit, alone."

I say, "How's it going?" He says, "Terrible . . . let me out of here." I ask him to tell me a little bit about himself. With a little coaxing, he tells me that he got married six months ago.

His wife is eight months pregnant with a girl. I ask him how he's feeling about all of this. He says, "I'm sick of it. I don't want to be married. I don't want to have a baby. I'm not ready for it. I'm a young guy. I can't go out, I can't do this, I can't do that. We're Catholic, she's very Catholic. . . ." So this pregnancy was a pain, which was a kick in the stomach for him. So there he was himself, pregnant as hell.

I said to him, "I think we can help you, but we're going to have to work on this, and you're going to have to cooperate by letting us explore this with you." Basically what I prescribed was talk therapy, and in about three days he was asymptomatic and went home.

So there it was. Within a week I had gone from the very trivial, with my friend and his skin tag, to a serious illness with hospitalization and a threat of procedures. That clinched my interest.

Getting into a cab on Second Avenue outside Bellevue, I felt completely removed from reality. My head was giddy, mostly with disbelief. How could this be? Can situations we normally think of as psychological be translated—or transduced, as Mack said—into physiological symptoms? Or, in other words, can a "psychological" state in a man produce symptoms in his body that mimic the physiological condition of his wife and partner? And what does it mean about the man? Does it mean he's happy about the pregnancy? He's unhappy? He's jealous? He's in synch? He's out of synch?

Next thing I know, there's a voice intruding upon my confounded thoughts. Great, yet another cabbie who wants to practice his English. It turns out that Juan is from Paraguay. Okay, so he wants to talk. I'll try out the "pregnant man" story on him. That will teach him a lesson, and buy me a quiet ride back to Brooklyn.

Juan from Paraguay chuckled and arched his eyebrows. "Have I ever heard of such a thing? Well, you know my brother had vomiting in the morning. What do you call it? 'Morning sickness,' thank you. Then he had toothaches, and so on and so forth. His wife used to joke that he was more pregnant than she was . . ."

Talk about transduction, as the miles pass I can feel the monotony of the road turn into relaxation, as some of the tension that I'd been storing up for the last six months oozes away. Soon we will be on the outskirts of Boston. We are on vacation! Our destination is Swan's Island, a small speck in the ocean off the Maine coast, where we will spend nearly a month.

As I drive Julie sleeps, her hand ever resting on her belly. Earlier we had been joking about whether this should be considered the last trip we have together as a couple, or to include the several billion cells that are Olivia, and call it our first family vacation. For a moment I have an image of her too, sleeping in her shockproof capsule, and an eerie sensation of carrying a third person in the car, until my guard dog brain cuts in and shoos Olivia away from personhood into the anonymity of the "fetus." I am not ready yet to think of us as three.

A few more boring miles and I realize how much I am looking forward to this trip. I've become a little sick of myself and my loopy behavior.

On the way up and back, we'll also be able to see our friends Matthew and Alice in Cambridge. Matthew and Alice are nationally famous for having lots of sex during their pregnancy. In fact, I think there is a shrine built in their honor on I–95.

In fact, I think I see it just ahead.

MONTH SEVEN

THE BODHISATTVA OF BIRTH

A fog-shrouded inlet, a cove
cupped in granite, the God-Mind's
vaporous pinkie paused in the geode
of the child-planet's teacup. On Swan's Island,
we are delivered into ourselves. Doubled over
your pregnancy, you peer through the viewfinder
into Earl Grey milkiness, your camera-mind blessed
with a momentary panorama of stress-free nothingness.
And mine, coursing the shoreline with labrador
randomness, is arrested with doggy wonder
at the eroded, abandoned armatures of dog-whelk,
urchins, periwinkles, and other minute hulks,
who lived to prove that time passes. I pray
what we have paused to reproduce blesses
us. That the signs we fail to see in this inlet's
sublime anagoge are already written into a sandy tablet
beyond, of some larger unseen felix mundi;

Growing now around the double-helix
Of our love, our part in the many-chambered future.

Sometimes being in a fog helps you see.

I'm thinking of those cloud-chambers I remember from my high school science books: gas-filled devices that enabled scientists to trace the path of subatomic particles, allowing them to study the hidden structure of all reality, the unseeable atom.

Ten miles off the Maine coast, Swan's Island sits in a cloud chamber. We've been coming to this craggy piece of rock for years. We rent an eighteenth-century cottage on an inlet for three weeks and get fundamental. There is nothing to do here— no bars, no restaurants, only one tatty little gift shop, and a general store with nothing in it worth buying. If you're one of the 300 permanent islanders, the main occupation is lobstering, as well as trying to preserve your sanity through the long winters.

A week has passed and the great internal spring of New York City life is almost slack. We spend our days enjoying the same little rituals, which in New York are reduced to mere ligatures. We talk. We fool around. We drink a lot of tea. We wander the shoreline aimlessly. Today, my mission was to find the world's smallest visible seashell. Julie snapped several rolls of film of fog. We cook—an endless supply of the freshest lobsters, crabs, clams, mussels, shrimp, and sea urchins are a moment away. We nap. Most of all, we read. I come equipped with a library of books and magazines. I read myself to sleep at night, and upon waking in the morning.

Here on this island without clocks, an opportunity to examine a self very different from the one addicted to the amphetamine of urban American life—a self I rarely see and can hardly describe emerges. A week on this island and your life's dream-state projector begins having bouts of mechanical apnea, occasionally sticking on the odd single frame. Luckily, this morning, that solitary stuttering image is beautiful. Lying in bed, head propped up on an elbow, I watch Julie comb out her hair by the bedroom windows which overlook Toothaker Cove. Backlit by a glowing scrim of fog, her belly, upon which the ends of her long hair rest, is a beautiful, soft sphere. Occasionally, a gust of air mixes the cheap gauzy curtains about her head.

While our bodies sag with relaxation, the feeling inside our cottage is fluid and weightless. I can finally see into my emotional interior, this uncharted, internal Bermuda Triangle I have been lost in for the last six months. Sadly, I see mostly anger. It's as if my psychology has been made physiological; as if the bars of my corporeal body have slackened, allowing my bitter, ranting doppelgänger to step out into the open light of the room.

What shocks me is the pettiness of these emotions. In the same moment that I finally appreciate the metamorphosis of Julie's body, I also realize I've been outraged over the physical changes. I feel as if I had a proprietary right to a certain image of her, as if I owned the copyright or the patent design. The naked indulgence of my objectification of Julie is bracing, embarrassing, but true. It may be irrational to feel this way, but it is not illogical. Pettiness shouldn't be mistaken for superficiality. The lack of subtlety in my reactions is telling. Emotions are fundamental and point beneath the gloss of cultural ideas and ideologies toward fundamental things. In this case, men do not like the bodies of their women messed with. But this is only the beginning. When I think back and trace the seemingly petty comments from friends like Adam, Gary, Joseph, and Robbie back to their roots, I could go on.

Men are divas. We simply don't know how to behave in stories where we do not play the hero. Pregnancy brings biological reality into conflict with a man's most important social feature, status. Pregnancy undermines our feelings of entitlement and the cultural stories that get us that entitlement. It threatens our most cherished privilege and reveals our dirtiest secret—our sense of authorship over our own lives *as well as* that of our partners. We sense the changing balance of power in our relationships with our partners, and anticipate the power they will hold over the life of the coming child and the future family.

Pregnancy for so many men of my generation signals a crisis. But why? The feelings that I just described are so contradictory. For most of human history, I can only imagine that a pregnant female would be a symbol of fecundity, of power for a man. What makes it so different today?

The short answer is symbolic. Pregnancy today, as well as much of parenting, occurs in a near symbolic vacuum for men, a void of ritual explanation, an absence of a place in a ritual story. One of the things that I feel almost physically, through my anxiety, is the complete divergence and disconnect between the *events* of my life and the *story* of my life. The events of my life are careering toward their destination like a bad car chase. The story of my life seems to be in freeze frame. (Kind of like trying to watch *Bullitt* with one mind's eye, and a Van Eyck still-life with the other.)

When you think about it, it's kind of insane. Pregnancy is perhaps our most powerful symbol of transition, of the potentiality of change. Yet pregnancy in our culture is a developmental transition without a script for men. Why, for example, do I feel like a bystander in the most important 280 days of my life? Where are the stories that make a man feel like he's in it, and not out of it? Where are the stories that help men and women negotiate the change in roles, status, and balance of power in partnerships? Where are the archetypal stories from which meaning descends to guide us through our more quotidian tasks and responsibilities? Where are the stories that help men emotionally manage the changes in their family structure? Where are the stories that create meaning? Where are these fucking stories?

I think the answer is simple. When it comes to stories of fatherhood, they are mostly gone. Somewhere, our culture discarded them.

Today I'm feeling relaxed. Today is the first day in seven months that makes me think I'm actually going to get the hang of this expectant father stuff. Today is also Julie's birthday, which makes all these good thoughts a potentially life-saving coincidence.

Since this is one of the few places in America without shopping malls I have been forced to be resourceful in the area of gift giving. This morning while she slept, I arose to write her a birthday poem. Then to Bea LeMoine's double-wide to pick up two pounds of fresh-picked crab meat. Later, to the general store to buy the makings of a birthday cake. In one of the aisles I managed to locate some boxes of Betty Crocker with expiration dates going back to prehistory. The mix must have gotten damp on the ferry trip over from Mount Desert, because the powder had turned to cement. Back at the cottage I had to hammer it back into rubble before I could bake it.

During the afternoon, we hiked a trail called Jacob's Ladder to the highest point on the island. There we scrambled—actually I scrambled while Julie picked her way gingerly—among blueberry bushes and rocks the size of boxcars. We caught our breath and ate our pack lunch with a 360-degree view of the Atlantic.

Later that evening for her birthday meal, I made crab cakes from an old James Beard recipe I found in a crumbling cookbook. One stick of butter per patty—Mr. Beard knew how to live. Our island friend Michelle and her lobsterman boyfriend Jason came over to join us. Afterward, I read Julie her poem and presented the cake, which had the loft and taste of oak planking. Oh well, it's the thought that counts.

Perhaps it was an optical trick, but when Julie bent over to make a wish, for a moment there was nothing but the sputtering of cheap candles and a little girl's face ringed in light.

Swapping mystery for knowledge hasn't done wonders for most of us. In most cases we have replaced mystery with what I call a proleptic fallacy—that is, we really don't have the "facts," but we anticipate science providing the "facts" in the "near future"—which is the same thing as saying that science has made us a society of control freaks. The problem is, life is basically still pretty mysterious whether you're a mystic or a materialist, but instead of acknowledging the power of the unknown and integrating our reaction to it into our lives, most of us are running around with placeholders in our heads: "To be dealt with in the future by science."

Science, while a blessing to our physical lives, is inadequate as a belief system. Why? The narratives of science, which have become the default ambiance of our culture—the *New York Times* has a weekly science section, not a weekly spirituality section—do not really address one of the most fundamental aspects of our biological character: Emotions form the core of our perception, and by far constitute the bulk of experience.

Often, the technologies that multiply our choices amplify our anxieties. Amniocentesis and IVF are blessings, but they do nothing to help us manage our expectations or the emotions surrounding choices. Couples look forward to test results with dread, not as a joyous opportunity to reduce risk. Couples undergoing IVF are usually as stressed out as terminal cancer patients, not ecstatic that their chances for childbirth are increased from nearly zero to at least 15 percent.

Replacing ritual narratives with scientific ones has created a vacuum. The metaphors that science chooses are not appropriate to who we really are. Treating our bodies and minds as machines has impoverished us in ways we can't explain. Why do we pay therapists to tell us what our symbolic life looks like? Why are we so attached to shopping, to brands and logos? Why are people who have been brought up in a secular fashion turning in increasing numbers to orthodox religions? Why did half a billion people "show up" for Princess Diana's funeral?

And why do these searches for meaning take the form of compulsions?

The situation for men is even worse. Men have been herded into smaller and smaller areas of symbolic activity. As a result, men have turned—I think, in desperation—to outsized spectacles such as Promise Keepers and Million Man Marches to tell them who they are. Mass rituals such as football, soccer, and car racing have become so very important, and as Michael Jordan's salary proved, no price is too high to pay for iconic vending machines.

If pregnancy is such a symbolically rich time, why are men so ambivalent, so confused? The problem with placeholders in our heads, the problem with mechanistic metaphors, the problem with mass rituals that resemble addictions is that real ritual narratives are lost. Ask any car salesman. Or ask any football coach or member of the clergy. Ritual narratives arose as symbolic guides for life, conveying information and direction, helping to manage the emotional turmoil and enormous stress of transformational states. Take them away and what you have is angry, confused, and frustrated people.

No one has been more disconnected, more desynchronized from the emotional content of experience than men. Men disappeared from the story of the family a long time ago with the onset of urban-centered, industrial life, both physically and ritually. Is it too much to believe that perhaps men suffer from this loss? In the transition to fatherhood, men might benefit from stories that are inclusive and encouraging the same way women benefit emotionally and physiologically from their childbirth culture. The absence of these ritual narratives for men might also play a part in the higher rates of infidelity, alcohol and substance abuse, and emotional and physical abuse noted in expectant fathers. When women make the jump from the technological world to the symbolic, transformational world of pregnancy, their men can't follow.

Men's "strange behavior" during pregnancy hints at the link between the symbolic and the physiological. Certainly stress triggers behavior, but what those behaviors articulate is something much more complex than can be explained by saying, "He's stressed." Part of the problem is that we don't have the categories and the language to "see" the behavior in a way that makes sense to us.

This language doesn't have to be flaky mumbo-jumbo. Real ritual narratives, I believe, are a synthesis of physiological, psychological, and social mechanisms. I would describe them as "bio-psycho-social phenomena," to borrow a phrase from Mack Lipkin's description of somatization. Their symbolic meaning actually helps synchronize the cognitive with the emotional and most likely evolved to help us deal with crucial developmental transitions in our lives. They are part of the way we try to connect with each other.

Trethowan had an inkling of this when he speculated that couvade syndrome occurred in cultures without couvade rituals.

(Couvade symptoms as a sort of an "illness" brought on by the absence of rituals.) Mack Lipkin, the researcher I visited who had done a study on couvade symptoms, noted that "in some cultures direct expression of emotions is permissible, in others it is not. When a culture does not allow direct communication of emotional content, somatization may serve indirectly to communicate psychosocial stress to others. In effect, patients somatize in accepted ways when direct emotional expression would be highly stigmatizing."

What Lipkin seems to be suggesting is that there is a direct, inverse relationship between ritual behavior and physiological behavior. Cultures that have ritual couvade provide an explicit script for men to negotiate their emotions and their expectations of childbirth and parenting. Following this reasoning, in Western societies, where male exploration of emotion is neither customary nor particularly acceptable, where male parental scripts are absent or unsatisfying, men express their fears, anxieties, or hopes about the experience of expectant fatherhood by having symptoms. The mind then uses the body to create a pathway for implicit emotional expression that is acceptable.

Physiological behavior is the equivalent of ritual behavior—the mind communicating through symptoms a symbolic expression of its internal state to other minds. And following this reasoning, my vomiting into the bathtub during Julie's first trimester qualifies as a poem written by my central nervous system.

I also think this link between symbolic communication and physiology can be stretched to cast light on the spontaneous rituals so many men make up during their wives' pregnancies. Look at the parallels between the "magico-religious" couvade rituals of preliterate societies and the rituals that modern men invent. Fathers restrict their diets, avoid activities to safeguard the health of the fetus, mimic birth pangs, and so on. Is that different from Jesse Nadelman, who monitored his wife's diabetic diet and restricted his own diet? Or from my best friend Gary, who allowed his precious testicles to be operated on to extract sperm, and was so obviously proud of the pain he went through? The craziest example I can think of is my friend Jerry, a former heavyweight boxer. Jerry claimed that he knew his wife, Carol, was pregnant before she did.

"Carol and I were at a cocktail party. I was camped out at the buffet table eating olives when I just felt something. I knew. I went over to Carol and told her to stop drinking. I told her that she was pregnant. She said, 'Jerry, you are so crazy!' Well, I was right. The next day she gets a test that confirms it. I immediately did a lot of reading and made up a special diet high in protein for her. I also put her on a light workout program, to keep her toned and fit. At night I would read stories to Carol's belly so that the kid would recognize my voice and know who I was immediately after she was born."

In the absence of explicit childbirth rituals, feeling stress, and faced with a life-transforming event, these men spontaneously created their own couvade to give themselves a place in the unfolding story. The *meanings* that these men derived from their behaviors helped them identify with the process. It gave them a sense of partnership, as well as a chance to bond and develop a relationship with the fetus on their own terms.

Just like hearing women's stories about childbirth, hearing men's stories about expectant fatherhood and their parallels with couvade rituals makes me wonder whether I'm hearing the echo of something ancient. Which brings me to a question: Are they relics like the abandoned, eroded periwinkle shells that make up the shores of Swan's Island? Or is it more like witnessing the flash of a something through the fog of our modernity—a universal and underlying reality that exists all around us? For the moment unseeable, but very much alive?

While Julie and I were packing to leave the island, I picked up a stack of reading material that I'd brought along and then assiduously ignored. At the bottom of the pile was *The Couvade and the Onset of Paternal Care: A Biological Perspective,* published in 1996. Beneath the eye-glazing title is an eye-popping premise. Robert Elwood and his coauthor Carolyn Mason, both researchers at Queen's University, Belfast, hypothesize that a man may have a physiological response during his partner's pregnancy that triggers a paternal behavioral change just prior to the arrival of the newborn.

Their reasoning relies on several factors. First are observations of behavior changes in the males of other mammalian species, including carnivores (lions), rodents (gerbils), and primates (langur monkeys), who are commonly infanticidal. Why? Because it benefits your genes. Imagine you are a Mongolian gerbil, or better yet, a male lion. *The Lion King* notwithstanding, killing young that are not your own means not having to waste energy raising young that don't carry your genes. It's also kind of an added-value meal. Most important, loss of young also causes the female to go into estrus, allowing you the opportunity to impregnate her. The resulting offspring would then carry on your genetic heritage.

Killing your *own* children, however, would not be advantageous. The question then becomes, is there a mechanism that allows males to distinguish between their offspring and the offspring of others?

Not a specific mechanism, but a generalized one. During their

mates' pregnancy, males shift from infanticidal or indifferent attitudes to a paternal state toward all young that they encounter, thus
ensuring the safety of their own offspring when they are born.
What causes the shift to this paternal state? Researchers have noted
what seem to be causal factors in a variety of mammals, the main
one being cohabitation and associated factors such as specific
interactions between male and female partners and odors given off
by the pregnant female.

Most fascinating, though, is evidence that suggests that the
onset of paternal care may be an expression of physiological
changes. In certain biparental mammalian species such as California mice and Mongolian gerbils, higher levels of prolactin
have been recorded in males just prior to the birth of their first
litter. In the biparental common marmoset, males with infants
were found to have prolactin levels five times greater than those
without infants. Levels of other hormones such as oxytocin,
vasopressin, and testosterone also may play a role in parental
attachment and behavior. For example, vasopressin injected into
the brains of male prairie voles has been shown to enhance
paternal response. Elwood and Mason conclude, "thus, a variety
of hormones, alone or in a combination, appear to influence the
paternal state of males of biparental species."

What does this have to do with humans? While, Elwood
explains, it is inappropriate to generalize findings from animal
to human populations, animal studies do provide a platform for
thinking about human behavior. There is plenty of evidence to
suggest that human males undergo a significant change in
behavior during the pregnancy period. Paralleling their reasoning with other mammal species, Elwood and Mason begin by
citing a detailed study of North American homicides that
showed a statistically significant, higher risk to children from

substitute fathers than from biological fathers. "That is, a new male entering the family unit is substantially more likely to harm the children than is the biological father, who has presumably lived with the mother since conception."* Obviously not all stepfathers are killers, but since a higher percentage of them do kill, what makes biological fathers less likely to be violent?

They pose a multidisciplinary argument to show that men do undergo behavioral changes, even though those changes are poorly understood. From anthropology, they cite ritual couvade as an indication of behavioral change. They cite psychological studies that have documented behavioral changes in men that been termed "pregnancy careers." From medical studies, Elwood and Mason then review and discuss the different studies of physiological couvade or couvade syndrome, noting the high incidence rates of symptoms in expectant fathers.

The bottom line? Plenty of evidence from both social science and medical science suggests that men have a significant and sometimes profound response to fatherhood, and that the commonly held medical view that men have a secondary form of relationship with the new child with no precipitating hormonal, physical, or emotional experiences is nonsense. The problem is, no one has given a satisfactory or convincing or testable explanation for any of the behavioral changes that take place.

Elwood and Mason propose such an explanation. How they do it is fascinating. Instead of viewing ritual couvade and couvade syndrome as separate phenomena, they view all men's behavioral change, whether ritual, psychological, or physiological, as part of a

---

*M. Daly and M. Wilson, "A Sociobiological Analysis of Human Infanticide," in *Infanticide: Comparative and Evolutionary Perspectives* (New York: Aldine Press, 1984).

continuum of effect, and propose a unifying cause. What could be the one thing that could tie social states, mind states, and body states together? Like California mice, or Mongolian gerbils, or lions, or langur monkeys, human males, in their estimation, undergo some physiological process that changes their behavior. This physiological process is then expressed as both couvade syndrome and ritual couvade.

"We suggest that the couvade syndrome in male humans is better explained as being due to physiological changes that mediate paternal responsiveness. That is, the various psychosomatic symptoms that constitute the couvade syndrome are a perception and interpretation of the normal processes in the male that bring about parental responsiveness. The couvade rituals seen in various non-industrialized societies may be a ritualization of the couvade syndrome. Ritual couvade may be better understood as a ritualized expression of underlying biological changes that function to bring about a state of heightened parental responsiveness. As in other animals, these biological changes in the male are likely to be triggered by the partner's pregnancy."

Bingo.

The ferry backs away from the dock, pulled, it seems, as much by the tug of our city lives as by its own engines. Swan's Island recedes into the distance, already a part of memory. At least we will take it easy on the way back, stopping over in Boston to see Matthew and Alice for several days. Against my better judgment Julie is driving the first shift. I have nothing necessarily against her driving, just that, having grown up in Manhattan and gotten her license at twenty-eight, she is not exactly a natural. Negotiating an I–95 onramp, for her, requires the mental preparation of a shuttle launch. So great is her anxiety that once she actually sought out the services of a hypnotist. After helping her visualize a calm and peaceful place, he told her to count backward from ten whenever encountering stressful driving conditions. However, sitting in the passenger seat and hearing Houston Control operating inside her mind isn't doing wonders for my nerves.

I set my spousal reassurance module on automatic and retreat inside to think over the consequences of Elwood and Mason's theory. Their ideas are risky. For example, they rely heavily on anthropological data, without taking into account the reliability of some of the sources of this data. Anthropologists are subjective. Interviewees may tailor their accounts to please interviewers. Cross-cultural interpretations of beliefs and behavior are difficult. Much of what is considered anthropology actually predates anthropology as a standardized discipline, and is often the second- and third-hand accounts of travelers. And so on.

The other potential liability is that they argue from animal behavior. Elwood and Mason themselves state that generalizing about human behavior from animal studies is inappropriate. But saying this is the same thing as flashing those "don't try this at home" disclaimers for bungee jumping or fire eating. Scientists don't want the general public to speculate because we may hurt ourselves, but the truth is that scientists speculate from animal behavior all the time, and proponents and opponents use similarities and differences in behavior between species to their advantage depending on what the argument is.

In Elwood and Mason's favor is a scientific and philosophical principle called Ockham's Razor. Named after William of Ockham, a noted fourteenth-century philosopher and heretic, this principle states that when there are multiple, competing explanations to a problem, the simplest, most elegant solution should be given priority. I remember having similar thoughts months ago when I was researching ritual couvade and subsequently stumbled across the references to couvade syndrome. Isn't is reasonable to speculate that there may be a connection between a ritual that has been reported for over 2,000 years in practically every corner of the globe, and a physiological phenomenon with startling high cross-cultural incidence rates? It seems logical to me to speculate that the two might be linked, and that a biological mechanism would be the most economical and most elegant premise to tie them together.

The only problem with Ockham's Razor is that it has two parts. The second part says that an explanation for an unknown phenomenon should first be attempted in terms of what is already known. Here, as I said, Elwood and Mason are on shakier ground. But in the end what truly favors Elwood and Mason is that their ideas are testable. If some sort of physiological paternal response mechanism could actually be documented in men, their speculative shack of cards could be transformed into a sturdy bungalow of hypothesis.

Speaking of shacks, we have stopped at a Maine version of a gasoline station-slash-convenience store, lobsters and deer heads nailed to the wall. Inside I buy some candy and every newspaper I can get my hands on, having been deprived for the last three weeks. Outside I find our little red Honda tilting heavily to starboard. Captain Julie, after filling the car, has used the principle of Ockham's Sledgehammer, having decided that the quickest route home was directly through a metal stanchion post located at the end of the pump island. The whole driver's side is bashed in. It's truly amazing the amount of damage you can do at three miles per hour.

I spend the next two hours buried in the *New York Times* catching up with the Summer Olympics, quelling an almost irresistible biological impetus toward uxoricide, and listening to a continual countdown toward possible oblivion.

Five . . . four . . . three . . . two . . . one . . .

So Matthew, exactly how much sex did you have during your pregnancy?

Yes, we had a lot of great sex when she was pregnant. I found it very liberating. For the first time in my life I wasn't ambivalent about something I was doing. It all goes back to that dream I had. It was the reason Alice and I were together.

If you met Matthew you would say to yourself, "Here is a man who works hard at keeping his house in order," and you would be right. Matthew, a practicing Buddhist, gets up daily at 3 A.M. for meditation sessions at a small shrine in the basement, before he heads off to work.

The Buddhists believe that all life is suffering, and for me getting up every day at that hour would significantly increase my suffering. It works, however, for Matthew. I do know that he has done his share of suffering, most of it self-inflicted. He is a person who has what used to be that quintessential of American qualities, "seeker," branded across his brow, which you wouldn't necessarily notice because most people who meet him are staring at his belly button. His brow rides about six feet, seven inches off the ground, just underneath a flash fire of red hair.

While Matthew cuts a Bunyanesque figure, much of his life has been spent trying to dismantle American myths, not create them. The son of a small-town doctor, he spent his youth as a member of the Revolutionary Communist Party, a Maoist group that spends most of its time in union organizing. He eventually left the RCP and a first marriage to another party member, and became a Buddhist.

Here in the heart of Cambridge, Matthew and his second wife, Alice, have built a life of deliberate balance. They have a different formulation on the American trinity of Work, Family, and Self. Matthew is the only American male I know who has repeatedly turned down promotions to keep things the way they are, and Alice's joke is that they are downwardly mobile.

(We're sitting around his kitchen table. I pour him another single malt whiskey.)

I was trying to do something right in my life. I had gone down a lot of different paths. After my first marriage blew up I had a lot of guilt. I tried going the monastery route, renouncing everything. I thought I could meditate for the rest of my life. But after a while, I had a bellyful of peace and idealized spirituality. I realized that I needed something real. I realized that having children was part of finding my way in the world.

It's funny, you know, I had a dream that winter, even before Alice and I started seeing each other romantically. We had just become friends. The dream was that I was here and Alice was there, and there was a child between us. I took it as a sign, as my own internal green light. If Alice and I were to get together, that's what it would be for. When Alice told me she was pregnant, I was unequivocally positive. It answered a deep unanswered need in me.

Alice actually was the ambivalent one, because it wasn't something we had planned. I immediately did everything I could to reassure her and her family about my commitment. I was going to stick around and be a partner and provide materially.

And the pregnancy itself? How did you handle it?

The pregnancy itself was a mess. I had ideas about natural childbirth, and I wanted to participate. Unfortunately Alice got sick. She had a condition called preeclampsia, or extremely high blood pressure, which is dangerous for both the mother and the baby. It was a rough ride. I wanted our birth to be an extremely personal process, and here we were in this teaching hospital surrounded by doctors and nurses. The medical students they brought in as observers were really the last straw.

May Lynn was born at seven and a half months. It was a very disorienting and intimidating experience. So many different people were handling her. It left me with such mixed emotions about the experience. In some ways I felt beholden to the technology because it potentially saved both Alice's and May Lynn's life. And then sometimes I think the midwives could have pulled her through on their own. It's made me wonder what's lost when technology becomes paramount. It was hard to get a human response from anyone. I ended up yelling in the delivery room for them to take the baby over to Alice before they took her off to intensive care. I didn't feel like I had any control over anything. It was like being on the outside of your own experience.

It seems so hard to imagine what existed before that technology was there. I think that ironically it reduces our own faith in our own capacities to respond to the demands of life, and that is a very serious thing. It is a metaphor that goes beyond birth. We are becoming so outside of ourselves. It's as if we don't have the equipment, the language to deal with our own experiences.

That's why it's important that these stories get told. Addie, one of the midwives who attended the birth, lives in our neighborhood. Whenever she comes over, we inevitably talk about it, the birth. It's part of what holds us together. It's the way we use language that makes us a community of people.

How did you get yourself through it? Did it change you?

You're going to laugh at me, Mr. Mystic and all, but I keep going back to that dream. It gave me strength to know why Alice and I were together. Not everyone has a structure or a story that gives shape to their lives. My spiritual practice gave me a metaphor to work with, the concept of the Bodhisattva, that enlightenment as well as self-benefit comes through relieving the suffering of others.

In the end, who knows why we have children? But this gave me the model to help Alice and to be an active parent, and my life experience gave me the story in which to act it out. Meeting Alice, the pregnancy, having May Lynn ... it was all part of a spiritual march, a process, and training. This was meant to be. This was part of my path. I needed to do it. And when I look back, maybe all of that goddamn inner work did some good.

With that we turned in for the night. It was late, and we had lost track over who was doing the actual talking, the whiskey or us. Three hours later I awoke momentarily. It was Matthew. I could hear him descending the stairs to his inner basement.

The importance of ritual and the power of its "meaningfulness" can be summed up in one word: "connectedness." If Elwood and Mason are right and ritual couvade was based on the foundation of physiological couvade, then there ultimately may be a symbolic communication between our body and our society that starts at the cellular level. Rituals may be, to steal a phrase from Mack Lipkin, "biopsychosocial" phenomena, a synthesis of physiological, psychological, and social mechanisms that help us deal with important developmental transitions in our lives. Couvade symptoms and couvade rituals are related on the symbolic level: Both indicate the need for men to communicate their internal states to their partners, their family units, and their groups.

This extreme need to communicate reflects how important it is for everyone that men manage the "crisis of pregnancy": the need to transform oneself when faced with inevitable transition. I am reminded of the Chinese ideogram for "crisis," which is a combination of the characters for "danger" and "opportunity."

On the side of opportunity, men can harness the transformative, symbolic power of pregnancy to make their relationships stronger and their lives more meaningful. Think of the stories we've heard. Jesse, the television cameraman, identified with his wife's experience—with the help of the metaphor of collaboration he brought from his work—and viewed the pregnancy as part of his own developmental transition to true adulthood. After a nine-inch canula was stuck into his balls, compulsive, hyperactive, career-mad Gary had a "birth experience" that forced him to connect with the meaning of his life, and allowed him to repair his relationship with Louise after his affair. Matthew? No wonder he was able to have a lot of sex. He felt comfortable. His dream of having children with Alice led him to feel that becoming a parent was an integral part of his spiritual path, which in turn allowed him to feel fully invested in his role as a nurturer for his partner and his child-to-be. With this metaphor, Matthew scripted a future for himself, putting behind him the questionable decisions of his past.

PREGNANT MAN

These men used the flux and transition, the symbolic power of pregnancy as an opportunity to rewrite the story of their lives. They reinvented themselves with their self-initiated couvade rituals. They took symbolic action in a way that allowed them to embrace the pregnancy as their own. They wrote themselves into a story that gave them a feeling of purpose, of participation, of direct connection with their partners and their soon to be children, and launched them into fatherhood and adulthood.

The absence of meaning also has its consequences, which brings me to "danger." Think of those men who got left outside their experience, friends like Robbie and Adam, whose ambivalence, anger, and other unresolved feelings about pregnancy spilled over into their marriages. Ironically, it was Adam the Shrink who remarked that many failed marriages can trace their dysfunction back to a pregnancy period, having fallen victim to the couple's inability to negotiate and forge new roles.

I think it's also important to realize that women have to consider their role in the process. Taking a tip from the Huoarani, couvade is a ritual for both partners. Pregnancy is a rite of passage and a developmental stage that requires both partners to make the crossing to social maturity. Partners need to experiment cooperatively to transcend the gender boundaries that confine pregnancy and parenting roles. I think of Joseph's complaints that Joan "took all of the emotional experiences for herself," leaving him marginalized. Women need to expand their thinking about pregnancy beyond their own bodies, and invite their men into their pregnancies in a way that is meaningful, making them "pregnant," too. And if men find themselves "written out of the story" during pregnancy, they literally need to find the right metaphor that they can use to write themselves back in.

•   •   •

The question I'm left with is, what will be my metaphor?

Being a science-loving atheist and not at all spiritually inclined, I can't really go Matthew's route. Besides, I have only two months left, hardly enough time to become an enlightened being.

A day later I have my answer. Matthew and I were indulging in the ancient male rite of lounging around in front of the television watching sports and drinking too much beer. All I can say in my defense is that it's the Olympics, not NFL football—although the difference is hardly discernible. The American athletes are so loaded down with sponsor logos that they should be given handicaps. And you would think that the fate of the free world, never mind a hundred million in endorsement contracts, rested on whether Michael Johnson would beat Frankie Fredericks of Namibia to become only the second man in history to win four gold medals. Poor Frankie. If I were he, I'd watch my back for gunmen on grassy knolls wearing Nikes.

There was, however, one moment of great authenticity. Jackie Joyner-Kersee, the two-time defending Olympic champion and world-record holder in the heptathlon, pulled up lame after the 100-meter hurdle event, practically collapsing with pain. All month she had nursed a badly strained hamstring, hoping to try for an unprecedented third heptathlon gold. Now, she sat on the apron of the track in tears hugging her husband and coach, Bob Kersee, who was speaking softly into her ear. Incapacitated with pain and with her health on the line, she depended on him to make a decision about whether she would continue.

I am not one for sports metaphors, but here was something I could relate to. There was something so validating about the two of them together in that moment of crisis. She was the athlete, but there was an obvious equivalence in their roles. He didn't do the running, but he was also not secondary. He was integral and essential to her success, both as a nurturing coach and a nurturing husband. It was so obvious that he had run every step of every race with her.

And there was also something else that was so clear—their personal partnership. Under the obliterating, impersonal gaze of national television, they transformed themselves from athlete and coach into wife and husband. It was he who had something unique to give. It was he to whom she turned to give her comfort and ease her suffering.

Could I not try to be Julie's Bob Kersee?

Suddenly, there were other things that I could see clearly. There was a flash and Bob Kersee turned into Matthew yelling in the labor and delivery room for the nurses to hand May Lynn to Alice. Another flash, and there was Gary on the operating table submitting to the nine-inch canula so that he and Louise could have a family. Another flash, and a Huaorani man was assisting his mother-in-law at his wife's delivery. Was there not something transcendent here in the efforts of these husbands? Were they not part of the Bodhisattva ideal?

Oh, one other thing. A momentary flare across the beery fog chamber of my mind. The camera panned up to the Olympic flame, which started speaking to me in Charlton Heston's voice about the great struggle, the endless open-ended question—the passing of the torch of what it means to be human.

I laughed out loud, startling Matthew. "I know why we have children, Matthew."

He looked up from his Budweiser with concern.

MONTH EIGHT

WETWORKS

BETWEEN SHIT AND PISS

Comparisons to orchids, lotus blossoms, and other literary floral arrangements seem somehow wholly inadequate once you examine a vagina from the distance of about three inches in decent light. What comes to my mind is a passage from Simone de Beauvoir's *Second Sex*:

> The sex organ of the man is simple and neat as a finger . . . but the feminine sex organ is mysterious even to the woman herself, concealed, mucous, and humid as it is; it bleeds each month, it is often sullied with bodily fluids . . . a horrid decomposition . . . Man dives upon his prey like the eagle and the hawk; woman lies in wait like the carnivorous plant, the bog, in which insects and children are swallowed up. She is absorption, suction, humus, pitch and glue, a passive influx, insinuating and viscous.

Lighten up, Simone. Actually, from a distance of three inches Julie's sex organ looks more like one of those undersea volcanic vents located in the deepest oceanic trenches that some scientists theorize gave birth to all life on the planet. What am I doing on this organic spelunking mission? I am journeying to the center of Mother Earth. I have rappelled down the ventral face of the goddess to check out her plumbing. With Julie's abdomen looming large above me, I feel very small in my maleness. For the moment, her organ is occult in its silence, but I am constantly on the alert for any seismic rumblings, gaseous venting, noxious spew, and any other life-giving but potentially unpleasant events. After all, my face is only moments away from most of Julie's major orifices. What is it that St. Augustine said? *"Inter urinas et faeces nascimur."* Between shit and piss we are born. Now, he was a happy fellow.

Guided by the light of my miner's lamp, I carefully reach into my utility belt, extract a Kleenex, and wipe away some white discharge on the labia. Satisfied, I then unfold a nearly illegible, Xeroxed sheet of instructions put out by some pathetically underfinanced childbirth education clinic. I can barely make out the letters, they are so crazed and crackled from endless duplication: Prenatal Perineal Massage.

It reads like instructions for a sixteenth-century appliance, although I am sure the Inquisition had better manuals. *Step one: wash your hands.* I'm a step ahead of you. Not only have I washed my hands, but I've also clipped my fingernails. *Step two: Find a private place and a comfortable position.* Okay, okay, as if we're going to do this on a park bench. *Step three: Use a lubricant, such as K-Y Jelly, cocoa butter, vitamin E oil, or pure vegetable oil on your thumbs and around the perineum. You can also use the body's own natural lubrication.* Huh? Natural lubrication? I've had quite enough of nature at this point. Let's go with the K-Y Jelly. We just happen to have some handy. *Step four: Place your thumbs 3–4 cm inside the vagina and press downwards and to the sides at the same time. Gently and firmly keep stretching until your partner indicates she feels a slight burning, tingling, or stinging sensation. Hold the pressure steady at that point for about 2 minutes until the area becomes numb.* Two minutes? At thirty seconds, Julie's mouth has oblated into the "O" in agony, protest, howl, and stop. I ease up, and give her a minute off. Getting to two minutes is going to take a while.

My mission here in the nether regions of the female anatomy is not pleasant, but it is necessary. After all, the soft mush under my fingers will eventually become the fleshly circle through which Olivia's head must pass—a circle stretched so taught it is known as the "ring of fire." The idea here is that prestretching the perineum, or the flesh between the lower vagina and the anus, will help the perineum be more elastic during the actual childbirth, helping to prevent tears, and reduce the need for an episiotomy. That's the theory.

Bizarre as perineal massage may seem, it's also the first thing in this whole pregnancy process that is working for me, that makes me feel useful. For seven months I have been looking for some common ground in this process, something that I can actually do besides being nurturing and supportive, something that—dare I say it?—is hands on, and I think I have finally found it. I feel relevant, I feel validated: My own experience of intense pain of long duration, and my self-taught methods of dealing with it give me something unusual and valuable to offer to help Julie prepare. My "coach" metaphor is not just an affectation.

Pain is something I understand. I have an intimate relationship with it from the three year-long injury rehabilitations I have undergone to the excruciating endurance sports—like long-distance cycling—that I love. Pain is also part of growing up male.

From the time you are a Little Leaguer and see a buddy catch a ball in the teeth, until you get carried off the high school football field with your leg sticking out at a weird angle, pain, acceptance of pain, tolerance of pain is ingrained as part of the wacky bushido of maleness. It makes me feel even better that this gift comes from me as a man as well as her partner—an offering from the gods of my sex to help her prepare for the thing she fears the most.

I also enjoy the strangeness of perineal massage. The idea that it is something few men would attempt, and I also suspect few women, adds to the allure of the experience, and to our own sense of intimacy and partnership. The other day I remember trying to explain it to my running buddies. We were cooling down after a run, sitting in Ozzie's, a favorite local coffee bar. They were razzing me for falling behind on the runs. Maybe it's the heat, or maybe I've just been feeling tired lately. Anyway, to change the subject, I started telling them about our perineal adventures. When I got to the part about my latest pudendal flesh stretching techniques, two of them could contain themselves no longer. A moment later iced coffee was spewing everywhere, and patrons were diving for cover.

Step five: Keep pressing with your thumbs, while slowly massaging back and forth over the lower half of the vagina for 3–4 minutes. When thirty seconds is agony? When I think of what it will take to work up to three to four minutes, an evil smile crosses my lips. All those arguments I lost over the years . . .

BIRTH PARTNER, BIRTH PLAN

Like a wandering husband who renounces his philandering and returns to his wife with a fresh eye, I now return to *The Birth Partner*, and the other childbirth manuals waiting patiently on my nightstand, with renewed commitment. One of the things I immediately like about *The Birth Partner* is that, lo and behold, it seems to be written for men, which at this point I really appreciate. It is straightforward, non-touchy-feely, economical with words. It is neither solicitous nor condescending. It tells you when to pay attention and why. It tells you when you can be useful, and when to stay in the background. It tells you all the important moments, who the players are, what they will be doing, and the risks. It uses charts and columns to lay out information. It is everything I remember lovingly about my high school football coach.

Going through the book together is a step-by-step way of being in synch on the major issues. One of the smartest things my friend Adam the Shrink said was, "Make sure you go into your pregnancy on the same page as your wife, make sure you are sharing the same story." Of course, in his own pregnancy experience, he promptly began to freak out. One of the first things *The Birth Partner* suggests seems deceptively simple: Pack a bag of supplies you'll need for the hospital. I say deceptively simple, because nothing between Julie and me is ever simple.

First of all, the bag. She picks up some cloth number with a crazy indigenous-type pattern from some Peruvian street vendor. I say no way. The closures and the straps are flimsy string. In my manly panic as I'm hustling out the door, I'll bust everything wide open. What we need is my purple, super-sized, Eddie Bauer gym bag. It's strong, rated for Mount Everest, spacious, and full of neat mesh this and mesh that to carry all our stuff. Yeah, but it smells like a gym bag. No, it doesn't, because I never go to the gym. It's ugly. Look, who's going to be carrying this thing anyway? Not you, you're going to be moaning and groaning and threatening to pass out. I'm going to be carrying the bag, and I'm not going to be seen in public with a granola-friendly, tree-hugger bag. I win. The gym bag is going.

After that's settled, what actually goes in the bag goes more smoothly. We go shopping together for fresh toothbrushes, toothpaste, lip balm, and lotions. We sort carefully through our favorite possessions to decide who our chosen companions on this journey will be. Julie packs a flannel robe and slippers. I throw in a light fleece sweater, since hospitals are cold. The book also recommends that I take a swimsuit in case I have to accompany Julie into the shower. Okay, I won't question it. In with the swimsuit. I throw in a couple of magazines for down times, and a fresh blank notebook and some pens. I also pack a couple of plastic water bottles with sip-straws, and, thinking ahead to the possibility of sleeping on a cold floor, a small, roll-up, foam mat.

Then there are the things for Olivia. As Julie packs them, I look on with the fascination of a child. In goes a small packet of newborn diapers, each no larger than a handkerchief. In goes her first outfit, a striped T-shirt. Next a pile of "receiving blankets." I have no idea what they are for, but we already have a ton of them. Finally, a little hat. It's the end of July and ninety-five degrees, but, who knows, maybe the baby will get cold?

In contrast, writing a birth plan is more philosophically complex, but less personally contentious. Birth plans have become important because of all the different philosophies about birth that exist, and because in hospital deliveries most of the caregivers are strangers. Well before your due date, you review the plan with your OB or midwife, and send the plan to the hospital for reference before you actually come in to deliver. It lets everyone involved in the mother's care know what her overall philosophy and end goal is, what her priorities are, and what procedures she is willing to accept under certain circumstances. Writing the birth plan together is also an important process for the partners. It gets them to talk over and agree on the major issues, and it thoroughly prepares the birth partner to be an advocate.

Anyway, that's the theory. At the moment, actually writing the birth plan seems so overwhelming. Julie and I have met a couple of times for the expressed purpose of talking over the various issues. So far these sessions have consisted of Julie bringing up a point and me staring off into space, occasionally making sounds that I hope indicate mental cogitation taking place. Some of the things are no-brainers. "Of course we want to avoid episiotomy if at all possible." Or, "In the event of any problems we would like to have as much consultation as possible."

Aside from that, who can really say? I can tell that even Julie is having the same problem. We make statements like: "I would like to have my husband present at all times, for any and all procedures" that seem a little unreal. Do we really need to say this? Would anyone really try to stop us from being together? "For the comfort of the baby, we would like to have dimmed lights in the room, and apart from any routine procedures as little trauma for the baby as possible." I mean, will the baby really care? And who would want to do more than the routine? "My husband would like to cut the umbilical cord after birth." Will I really want to do that when the time comes? I don't really know; I've been told it's a wonderful thing.

That's the problem, you see. All the statements we are making propitiate two deities. One, a goddess of our ideal, inner experience, an experience we've been told that we should want, and that will put us in touch with our lost humanity. The other, an impersonal god of precision that promises absolute safety—a god that I've grown up with and, I have to say, often feel more comfortable with.

Finally, there is the unthinkable. "If I am unable to make certain decisions, my husband knows my wishes and should be consulted." "In the event of a stillbirth, we would like to have time alone with the baby and would welcome an opportunity to talk with a counselor." Frankly, neither of us really knows what we want in this situation, but that is what the book tells you to say. And that is why you read books. To trust those that have gone before to know.

Through all this there is one thing that serves as a point of reference and comfort. It is the purple gym bag that I have parked on the way to the door. Its presence means that there will be, finally, an end to this state of anticipation and unknowing. The earliest sign of an experience I can only hope will be incorporated later—after the doctors, the nurses, and midwives are forgotten—into our private book of happiness.

After all, it is packed for three.

CHILDBIRTH 101

The secret to childbirth education is to wear really great socks. Why? Because the first thing I've noticed about "CE"—as the instructors love to refer to it—is that you spend a lot of time with your shoes off and your socks showing. And if you can tell a lot about a person from his shoes, you can tell even more from his socks. Mine are frayed and showing through in places.

There is also nothing that levels the adult playing field faster than sitting around together on gym mats, shoeless, with your socks *en pleine aire*. My consoling conclusion is that Henry Kravis or Ronald Perelman or Rupert Murdoch for all their billions would look as silly in their socks as I do.

The other great leveler, of course, is abject fear.

A dozen of us pregnant couples are gathered in a drab studio somewhere in midtown. All the women are in the latter stages of the third trimester, and as I scan the room it's amusing to see how pregnancy is expressed throughout a range of physiognomies. Tall girls who are unchanged except for a bit of luggage low in the trunk. Fat girls who have turned mountainous. Tiny girls who actually seem to be attached to something larger than themselves.

We are all first-timers and our fear is obvious. If I were to be flippant, I would describe it as a supernova cousin of that feeling of group panic you had in fifth grade when you discovered that there was going to be a pop quiz and no one studied. But there is none of the levity—the chitchat, the camaraderie associated with assured, mutual, but nonlethal failure. Here, we all keep to ourselves and the air is viscous with anxiety. The women move with dreamlike, glycerin deliberateness, mostly to drink continuously from ubiquitous water bottles. Watching them, I keep thinking of potted plants, and wait expectantly for the overflow to dribble from their bottoms. The men are universally blank and passive, dead space in the guise of physiology. They seem to have all placed their brains in "park." The only animated beings in the room are the fetuses. Olivia seems to be in the middle of a channel crossing and is kicking up a storm, and judging from the frequent flinches from the other women in the room, she is not alone.

When our instructor, Erica, asks us to introduce ourselves and talk about our feelings about the coming experience, things perk up a bit. As we go around the room, one can almost see the demons scrambling to their cranial cockpits and the coping mechanisms burst to life.

"I'm afraid that my baby is going to be too big." "I'm afraid that I'm not able to be able to handle the pain." Then there are a few HMO-related concerns. "Eight months into my pregnancy and I don't even know where I'm going to give birth yet. The HMO's hospital doesn't have midwives, and I'm still waiting to hear whether they'll cover a delivery at the hospital where I'd like to deliver."

One couple gamely tries humor: "We're running low on amniotic fluid, so we're looking at the possibility of an early C-section. So if anybody has some extra to spare, we'll gladly accept."

Another couple comes prepared with a mission statement. From the "information is control" school, they seem determined to overcome their fear by turning their competitiveness on it. She says something like: "I've done a lot of reading and I'm committed to having a vaginal delivery without painkillers." He says something about "being more concerned with contingencies and high-risk scenarios." Sure enough, they're both lawyers.

One honest soul finally says, "I'm just really terrified. I've never done this, I've never seen it done. I'm just really scared."

Everyone nods. Elegantly put. Dittos all around.

Erica's reaction to all this is curious. I don't really know quite what to make of her. Here in Manhattan where you associate women with power suits and black cocktail dresses, she seems homespun in her jeans and hiking boots. Her speech is sprinkled with strange, vaguely New Age locutions. Everything is about "finding the place you need to be." About "honoring your body and honoring your birth." About "being in your experience." What do these words mean? And how is she going to keep the attention and gain the respect of a bunch of "I'm scared out of my mind yet still smarter than thou" New Yorkers?

Of course, silly me, what I had failed to consider was that Erica dealt with the likes of us all the time. For it was a few moments into her opening monologue that she emitted the sound that cleansed our minds of all doubt. It started as a low spongy moan, grew in intensity to a chthonic howl, flattened out into a primordial bellow, and finally tailed off in a rattling sigh—pretty much summing up the entire tragicomic trajectory of human existence. No doubt this was the sound that Adele Quested heard at the Marabar Caves.

Now that she had gotten our attention, she continued. "That's what birth really sounds like. You have to forget all of the media images of birth that you have been exposed to—you know, where the woman lies on her back in a squeaky clean, high-tech environment, moans a few times, and pops out a squeaky clean baby. They are not helpful. Also not helpful is the idea that women's bodies were not made to do this. Let's try a little experiment."

Erica quickly went around the room and asked how each of us was born, and how our siblings were born.

"I want you to consider this. A woman's body is a safe place to birth a baby. Just in this room alone we've have a history of sixty vaginal births with only three C-sections, and judging from the descriptions, two out of those three were probably unnecessary. What does this show us? Birth works. Our bodies work. They were made to make babies. The idea that your baby is too big for your pelvis, known as cephalo-pelvic disproportion, is a myth propagated by the medical profession. Most of us will grow a baby that is right for our pelvic opening.

"You also have to understand that every birth experience is unique, individual. Your birth experience will be unlike any other. But even though it is your very own experience, you are not in control of it. The pregnancy is a metaphor for the birth. You don't grow the baby, you don't get to pick the day, you're not in charge of this time frame. Only 3 to 5 percent of women actually deliver on their due date. It might take one person twenty hours to get to four centimeters, and another person, two. Here, let's try another experiment."

Again Erica went around the room, this time asking, "What is the shortest birth you've ever heard of?" Thirty minutes. (Room gasps.) The longest? Fifty-six hours. (Room gasps.)

"Look at the difference in experiences. Each birth is different because each body is different. Birth is not a script. It's much more like jazz. You have to adapt, and improvise. The starting place here is to be in your own experience, because it will be different than anyone else's."

To show us what real birth looks, sounds, and feels like, she popped a videotape into the VCR and turned down the lights. The first birth was a home birth, but it looked like it was taking place in the middle of a supermarket aisle. There were people everywhere. Not only was the woman's husband present, so were the rest of her kids. There also seemed to be a larger than normal contingent of birth attendants milling about.

Laboring Woman #1 was on all fours, "vocalizing," that is, emitting these moaning-roaring sounds. In the background of the audio track some lugubrious women's empowerment narration was droning on and on. A head shot of the laboring woman being interviewed was superimposed over the scene: "I felt like a tigress. It felt like all of the power in the universe was inside of me." The head shot faded away and the woman finally gave birth, the blood-flecked, mucus-slick baby sluicing out into the midwife's arms. Onscreen, the woman's family cheered.

Erica stopped the tape and turned up the lights. When I looked around the room, most of us wore constricted grins of relief. Mr. and Mrs. Mission Statement looked concerned. None of us had been ready for the raucous candor of the scene, nor the powerful, complex emotions it released, not to mention the enormous amount of bodily fluids. Someone blurted out, "It was so chaotic! How could they stand it?"

In response Erica asked: "Is anyone here going to have more than just their partners and their doctor or midwife at the birth? Nobody? We have a very private image of birth today, and the medical profession has tried to limit the number of people at the bedside. But traditionally, birth was a communal event, part of the life of a whole village or community. The woman you just saw chose to have her whole family there, as well as a massage therapist, a herbalist, and an acupuncturist. Having these people present can give the laboring woman an enormous amount of emotional and physical support. For example, having a labor doula has been shown to reduce the need for pain medication, as well as the rate of C-sections."

Birth #2 was a hospital birth. This woman was obviously in trouble. Hanging on her husband's shoulder, she looked distraught; her husband, concerned. As the video proceeded, she became increasingly laden with equipment. First, it was an external monitor. Then, an internal monitor. Next, an IV drip. Finally, most of the above, plus an oxygen mask and an epidural lead. Her tone on the voice-over was weary. "It took me forty-eight hours just to get to three centimeters. Then things just stopped. The doctor said, 'We can either do the C-section now, or I can do it in three hours,'" meaning I could try some more on my own, but the result would be the same. It made me so mad. They gave me an epidural and some pitocin. Ten minutes before the scheduled C-section they checked me again. The resident said, 'She's dropped,' and the nurse said, 'Okay, push, honey.' Half an hour later, my baby was born. Looking back, I have to say that the epidural turned out to be a good thing for me."

Even in the relative dark, I could tell that people were having a hard time with Birth #2. There were a lot of couples holding hands. Some wives curled up into their husbands' arms. There was also a lot of head nodding at the epidural statement from Woman #2.

"Now that's what I call a good use of an epidural and pitocin," Erica said, turning up the lights again. The epidural let her sleep, and the pitocin helped her body open up. When she woke up, she went through a fundamental shift in attitude, she was in a different place. She stopped trying to 'do' labor. She relaxed into the labor. She let go.

"In the interest of giving you different images of the birthing experience than you might have or the medical profession might want to give you, I want to spend a moment and talk about the situation she was in. The most frequent reason for C-sections is fatigue and sleep deprivation. There could have been very viable alternatives to pain medication and pitocin that could have helped her, but were ruled out by the hospital setting. For example, if this were a home birth or a birthing center birth, she would have been able to try any number of alternatives to try and get rest. A shot of vodka or a glass of wine. Herbs such as skullcap. A warm bath and a massage. And for some, medications such as stadol."

Birth #3 was also difficult. It was the woman's third birth. Hers was a "posterior baby," who had become hung up somewhere in the birth canal. The woman was trying out a variety of different labor positions in an attempt to "shake the baby loose." One moment she was on her hands and knees. Another scene had her kneeling, with her arms around her husband. Another, had her sitting on a toilet, vocalizing in great moans, her head in her hands. Yet another, relaxing in a tub. Finally, she gave birth with a great gush of blood and an enormous collective sigh of relief from our class. Who knows how long ago the actual birth took place and when the videotape was made? No matter. What washed over us was immediacy—the enormity of her effort and her eventual triumph. Great tears were rolling down my face. As I looked around the room, grateful for the darkness that hid my emotion, ditto everyone else.

"A couple of comments," started Erica. "This birth shows you how important it is to get rid of all of those images of women lying on their backs to give birth. This woman had a very difficult birth, but she was a very experienced mother and after trying a variety of positions she found what worked for her and this particular birth. I myself gave birth to my last child in the shower hanging on to my husband's shoulder.

"If you listen to women who have had many children, they speak like athletes about the experience. These people are very much in their bodies. They have a dialog with their physicality. The thing to do is to try and get to that place when it's your first time. And that's going to be my job, to help you get there. See you next week."

As we all got up to leave, all of us simultaneously looking for our shoes, I had the sense that the others felt as we did—this had been a transformative experience for everyone. But the question in my mind was, why so late in the game? If only this type of learning process had started early in the pregnancy, would we have all felt better? For that matter, why didn't someone teach us these things in high school biology? I couldn't help thinking about what Erica had said about birth once being a communal event. For all we say about our vaunted information revolution, how tempting it is to say how little we know about what really matters. And as we filed out the door together, I thought about the most horrible legacy of our modern lives and the epiphany I once had during a therapy session. Why is it that we always have to pay cash money for the knowledge that others feel as we do? That we are not isolated, not alone with our fear and our human suffering?

SERGEANT ROCK

I'm standing in the lobby of the Lenox Hill Hospital looking upon a scene of near-riot conditions, if you can use such a term to describe the behavior of rich pregnant women dressed in expensive maternity clothes and pearls.

Let me back up half an hour to the cause of all this fuss. Today Julie and I finally took a tour of the birthing facilities. We had been looking forward to this moment. At Seventy-seventh and Park Avenue, Lenox Hill Hospital is situated among some of the priciest real estate on the planet. We even got a little dressed up. Somehow, I had thought to have our birth experience among such luxe surroundings—courtesy of our OB's Upper East Side practice—would give us a leg up in the world. Surely, if the rich aren't treated with respect, who is?

Alas, one of the things you can say about the medical profession: It is more democratic than most of our institutions when it comes to mistreating people. Two problems became immediately apparent. One was the personality of our leader, the nurse conducting the tour group. She may be a competent professional, she may even be a good person, but her social skills are on par with those of Sergeant Rock Fury.

The other problem is the facilities. The half dozen or so labor rooms are about the size of barn stalls. There is also a delivery room, which is a much larger space with a birthing bed in it, a private bathroom, and a shower. But, as I said, there is only one of these. So if your cervix gives you the green light while the delivery room is occupied, guess what, you have to deliver Princess in the manger.

Problem #1 and Problem #2 converge when Sarge informs us that we, meaning the laboring parties, are expected to stay in the labor rooms until we are called to go to the delivery room. At one point, I think I actually hear her say the word "whining," as in "I don't want to hear any . . ."

On the elevator ride down, the fury is kinetic. The doors open and women wearing Donna Karan Maternity are swarming toward the public phones in the lobby. Another minute and they are all yelling at their OBs. One of them cries, "I want the delivery transferred to St. Luke's."

Julie and I look at each other. Has our birth plan just become a battle plan?

LABOR WHAT? NO, LABOR WHO

"A labor doula," Julie replied.

"What's that exactly? It sounds vaguely familiar."

"Weren't you paying attention in class?"

"Is this a pop quiz? I was more fixated by the part where your uterus has expanded to fill 75 percent of your body cavity, constricting your bladder to the size of a Chicken McNugget. Your eight trips a night to the bathroom are ruining my quality of life."

"I think we really need the help."

"The two of us aren't going to be enough?"

"Do I really have to answer that question?"

"No."

"Something happened the other day that convinced me."

"Oh?"

"I sat next to some women with young infants at the bagel place on Seventh Avenue. We started chatting, and they asked me all kinds of questions: When are you due, where are you delivering, has it been an easy or a difficult pregnancy, the usual. Finally, when I got up to go, they said, 'We'll be seeing you around.' It was something about the way they said that, something about their manner, and the way they treated me. It was as if there was a wall between us. As if there was an experience, a trial, a passage that they couldn't articulate, but that separated us. Whatever it was, I realized then, it was huge. And I'm convinced that we need someone there."

"How do you experience pain?" Susan, the labor doula, asked Julie.

"Well, I tend to internalize and withdraw, to get really quiet and curl up somewhere. When I have really bad period cramps, I sometimes roll up into a ball on the bed," Julie replied.

"How about you, Gordon? How do you experience pain?"

"Huh, who me?"

I decided that I was going to like Susan. In a quiet and gentle way, she got right to the point. No wishy-washy, fuzzy-wuzzy, loosey-goosey, feel-goodisms. She just came out right out of the box and tackled the 800-pound gorilla.

When Julie brought up the idea of having a labor doula at the birth, I didn't go for it immediately. I am a typical enough male in that I've had the "no, I don't need to ask for directions" syndrome ever since I was a newborn. It wasn't that I was exactly resistant—I just felt that I had little enough to do as it was, would this completely reduce me to the level of a token presence?

Like I said, male reasoning. But I quickly got over it. If Julie had reservations, with all the effort and study she had put in so far, who was I to feel comfortable or confident?

The experience at the hospital had definitely spooked us. Afterward, Julie questioned our whole approach and openly wondered whether we should have started out in the beginning with a midwife. No matter how competent in practice the medical professionals were—as Dr. Spyros, our OB, later tried to reassure us when we herded into her office to complain—the larger system just didn't have a place for the emotional state of the clientele. It even made us doubt Dr. Spyros herself. We had a good relationship with her. We felt she understood the type of experience we wanted, or at least preferred. We even felt that she was personally committed to try and help us achieve that experience. But we couldn't help but wonder; after all, she herself was a product of the same system.

In the end we decided it was too late in the game to switch. We would go forward with our plans, but adding a labor doula would at least give us a middle ground we were comfortable with.

"Yes, I was wondering how you experienced pain?" Susan repeated.

"Well, when I've had no other choice, I've tried to integrate pain, accept it as part of the experience. Instead of trying to shut it out, or shut down my mind, I actually try to let the pain in. Sort of take its measure, as it were, and treat it as a companion."

"Have you ever seen Julie in physical pain?"

It took a moment to remember it, but there was a time Julie and I went bike riding together in the intensely hilly country around her parents' country house in Connecticut. For those of you who are unaware of the pleasures of serious, high-performance road cycling, it is excruciating, a sport for people who love suffering. Julie is not a sportive person, but I had encouraged her to get her own bike and accompany me on some easier rides. One weekend, while visiting her parents with my best friend Charles, the three of us went for a ride. At one point, on the way back, we realized that we would have to climb a steep, three-mile grade. For Charles and me it was no problem. For Julie it was going to be a challenge. I thought she would have to get off and walk it, but she chose to gut it out.

There is a reason that the villain in the movie threatens to torture the girlfriend and not the hero. It is very difficult to watch a loved one suffer. The ride up the hill seemed to take forever. Charles and I took up our stations around Julie. I call out, "Breathe, breathe, breathe," in a rhythmical pattern, like a coxswain calling cadence for his oarsmen. Charles, a more profound explorer into the darkest regions of physiology than even myself, says in a quieter voice, "Smile at your inner organs . . . they are your friends." Grimace by grimace, revolution by revolution, we talk her up the hill. When we crest the top and the earth mercifully flattens out, Julie breaks out into tears and Charles and I let out a great cheer. It was a great moment. We never tried it again.

"Well . . . there was one time . . ." I told Susan the story.

"That's great," she said. "I think it's really important that you've had this experience together. It's something to build on, and I think it's going to be something you can refer to during the birth."

Susan went on to describe how she saw her role during the birth, and as she spoke we felt more and more at ease. She had attended more than a hundred births. She would be there from beginning to end for our birth, and her philosophy was not to force herself on the situation, but to help if needed, or stay in the background if that was more appropriate.

After the initial back-and-forth was over, Susan asked to take a tour of the house. "Think about where you want to spend the early part of your labor. Remember that one of our goals is to spend as much time as possible here at the house, not at the hospital. Think about the places that make you most comfortable."

Susan's request made us think about our apartment in a entirely new way, most of it negative. How could such a momentous episode in our lives start out in such prosaic and dingy circumstances? The bathroom was way too small. When Julie sat on the toilet, there wasn't enough room around it to get near her. The bedroom seemed dark and cavelike, in a word depressing. I made a mental note to myself: Remember to move to the suburbs as soon as possible.

We finally settled on the kitchen. It's relatively light and airy and has a view of the garden. We tried out several positions. Julie sitting on a chair. Julie hanging on my shoulders, while Susan massaged her back. Then Susan had Julie practice vocalizing. She started tentatively at first, a few perfunctory "oh-oh-ohs," until Susan stopped her. "That's not a bad start, but try to reach down deeper. Don't feel inhibited. This is really going to help with the pain. Take a deep breath, exhale with the sound, and make it loud enough so that you can feel it throughout your body."

Julie went for it—big, high-volume, elemental exhales that churned the molecules in my teeth.

Was this sound really coming out of my little Julie? I could hardly believe it. In between worrying that the neighbors would call the police to find out who was dying, I had the feeling of being transported forward in time. A jump-cut to the scary inevitability of the future. My eyes brimmed, and I ducked into the bathroom to be alone for a moment with my unwanted emotional nausea. Sitting on the toilet to collect myself, I, too, took some deep breaths and examined my feelings of powerlessness. Part of me wanted to stop the whole process, part of me wanted to take Julie's place—neither of which I could do.

I felt irrational. What can I say? I'm a man. I don't particularly like my emotions.

"Everything okay?"

I was walking Susan to the door. I followed her out to the street to chat for a moment. I liked her. She was making this whole thing feel real. "Yeah, thanks for asking. Most of the time I feel pretty much in synch. But there are times it's all a little overwhelming."

"It's only normal. And otherwise, how are you feeling in general?"

"Worried about me?"

"No, but I'm always interested in finding out how the partner is doing, as well as the mother. It's a team effort."

I thought about it for a moment. "You know, it's funny that you ask. I have been tired a lot lately. The other day I went for a run, and I almost stopped, I wanted to quit. It was a weird feeling. I never quit." I laughed. "Maybe I'm having pregnancy symptoms. Did you know that some men have symptoms?" dragging out my little factoid.

"Don't all men have symptoms?" Susan responded. She smiled and walked away and up the street. I watched her until she disappeared around a corner.

Quirky woman, that Susan.

THEM IS US

I'm not saying it's like John Carpenter's *Them*, where with the aid of special sunglasses the hero can detect the hideous aliens who are assuming the guise of humans, or even *Invasion of the Body Snatchers*, where Kevin McCarthy is trying to save a world increasingly populated by pod people, but men with couvade syndrome walk among us and in relatively large numbers. Like many other things in human perception, when you're not look- ing for it, it could be right under your nose and you'd never know. If you are looking for it, you see it everywhere.

One night while escaping my life by going onto the Internet, I ran into these postings on Parent Soup, a parenting Web site:

My DH [dear husband] has had more symptoms than me—he is ill in the mornings and wakes up in a sweat 5 times every night after dreaming awful things like the baby being born without a head. I am seriously considering my sister or a girl friend for a birth partner—I don't think he'll cope!

Finally someone else. My DH gets morning sickness for the first tri. In fact that is usually how we find out we are pregnant (this is my 3rd due in June). He starts getting sick in the mornings and then I go to the doctor. He gets violently sick. He ends up getting medication from the doctor.

My DH has been having sympathy "pains" too. On the days when I feel big, he feels bloated. Just yesterday he came home from work and said, "You feel big, don't you?" I couldn't help but laugh. He also gets moody, weight gain has been a definite problem for both of us, and yes, he has dreams about the baby too. But it seems like the more we talk about the baby, the easier it is for both of us to deal with all of the "wonderful" aspects of being pregnant.

Thank you—I will show DH these messages tonight. I always thought he was extremely perceptive of my feelings but this is amazing—I quite like it though—it's a pity he couldn't go through it all for me.

The idea of men having pregnancy symptoms is such a joy to me! I think it's wonderful when a man and woman really connect in this special way during pregnancy. Both nauseous, both bloated, both tossing and turning their nights away. Talk about a bonding experience.

Stumbling across personal reports of couvade syndrome is one thing; getting a chance to talk to men who have experienced it is another. The women trading these e-mails were comfortable talking to one another, but not necessarily talking about it to anyone else. When I posted a message asking for contact information I never got a reply. How was I going to get the chance to do an actual interview? Finally one day I mentioned the subject to a buddy of mine. He started laughing. "You've got to talk to my friend Derek."

Derek wasn't exactly thrilled to talk about his experiences. Couvade syndrome did not exactly fit Derek's idea of manhood. He's a twenty-first-century man's man. A hedge fund manager who splits his time between Martha's Vineyard and St. Bart's, he is into extreme sports. Skiing "off-terrain." Surfing in hurricanes. Sailing in typhoons. Downhill mountain bike racing. And then to relax, deep-water scuba diving. I shudder to think what he needs to do to make something like sex interesting.

After a little coaxing, I was able to find out a few things. "The two girls are three and four. The first pregnancy was much more symptomatic. The second one, I didn't feel as physically involved. I gained a few extra pounds, but that was it. The first time we didn't know Ally was pregnant right away. She was tired a lot, I was tired a lot. Then we found out."

And the rest of the pregnancy? What was that like?

I definitely had several periods of extreme fatigue. Early on I had morning sickness. I also had this weird kind of dietary synchronicity. We both had cravings at the same time for the same foods.

What was your labor and delivery like?

The worst part of the experience. I admit it, I'm a control freak. I found labor awful, and I think it's a huge mistake to have men present at the delivery. I think it's a cultural affectation. I mean, men have only been present during the last thirty years. There was nothing I could do except worry. The moment of birth is phenomenal, but most of the time the man just stands around. We're just not constructive to the process. Women are just a lot better equipped to deal with it than men.

Has fatherhood changed you?

I'm obsessed with not wasting time, whether I'm working or playing. I have these fuckheads calling me all of the time pitching stocks and companies. If I don't like what they're saying within the first thirty seconds, I hang up on them. Having kids has definitely taken the edge off me. I'm in love with my daughters. I used to like jumping off the edge of cliffs, now I just want to take them shopping for shoes.

My second interview was a breakthrough, a real corker. I had heard about Todd through friends of mine at a cocktail party. I had been talking about medical couvade when one woman started cackling, "You've got to talk to Todd."

Todd and his wife, Abby, also have two daughters. "I had it less the second pregnancy than the first. The first time I really noticed what was going on. Actually Abby pointed it out. I came home from work one day and I felt weak. My whole body ached . . . and I thought I was coming down with something. There was nothing I wanted more than a cup of tea, and I don't drink tea. I'm a coffee drinker. But I just had this incredible craving for tea. I associated it with when I was sick as a child and my mother would make me weak tea and toast.

"Anyway I said to Abby, 'I feel delicate. I can feel my skin. I feel like I'm coming down with something,' and Abby said, 'but that's how *I feel*, and tea and toast is what *I want*!'

"So we started comparing symptoms, and at that point I realized that I had morning sickness. We had not discussed this before; she had not told me what she was going through. I didn't throw up like she did, but I felt different. Something wasn't right, my body wasn't reacting the way it normally did. This was just six weeks into the pregnancy. It was so unexpected. It wasn't a case of 'Oh, I've heard of symptoms.' I'd never heard of this before."

What happened after that? Did you have any other symptoms?

I had a mirror pregnancy. It was so parallel that it was like "Okay, what's happening today?" I'd be the one to tell us what was going on, what we were feeling. My feet got flatter. I couldn't stand up for long periods of time. Lower back pain was the other really severe reaction. I couldn't sleep on my back anymore; I had to sleep on my side . . . I couldn't lie on my stomach.

Oh, yeah. We even started looking alike, which isn't easy seeing how I'm six-five and she's five-one. Since her body was changing she couldn't fit into her own clothes. So she started wearing mine, because they are bigger. So that got a little strange. We would buy things for her but I would have to like them because they'd become mine. So we kind of shared our pregnancy. In fact I really felt that I was pregnant."

How did that feel?

It was embarrassing. We didn't really talk to friends about it, afterwards because I was so totally embarrassed by it. It seemed so totally selfish in a way.

Why selfish?

To talk about it would be to make myself more important than I presumed I should be. It would detract from the "Mother," the "One Who Is Pregnant," the "One Who Is Going Through the Experience," the "One Who Is Going Through All of the Hormonal Changes." But I'm also a great believer in the idea that men have periods, too. I don't know exactly when they are, but I know when I'm having one. If you made a study of it I think you'd find that men have cycles.

So did this synchronicity with Abby make you feel part of the pregnancy or not?

Both. At times it made me feel closer to her and the process. Other times I felt very much the sidekick. I had one great fear. I had this idea that Abby would hate me when she was actually giving birth. That I would just be in the way. You hear these stories about women cursing out their husbands, "You did this to me." But it didn't happen.

What did happen at the delivery?

It took a long time. Abby's water didn't break and she didn't let them break it. At that point I'm not in control. I'm having doubts. I don't know whether she's in touch with her body or just being obstinate. The professionals are saying, 'We should break her water.' The doctor was insisting and insisting and insisting, until finally he and Abby were yelling at each other. I was thinking, oh my God are we doing something wrong? As it turned out she was right and he was wrong. She was able to say to him, as I wanted to, "You've never had a baby, you don't know what it was like. You've delivered them, but you don't know what it's like."

Sounds like things got way too dramatic.

Well, I have to tell you that the most dramatic thing that happened to me was after the delivery. It's kind of graphic and its kind of gross.

That's okay. Go ahead.

Immediately after the baby was born, we went to our room to rest. We were both there with the baby. It was less than an hour, when boom! I hadn't realized that for a week prior to her delivering—and she delivered a little late—I had not had a bowel movement. I wasn't in pain, I just hadn't thought about it. Anyway, I had the largest dump in human history. It was unbelievable. I kept calling into the room to Abby, "It keeps coming and coming!" It was enormous and it hurt! It had to weigh more than the baby. Yet there was something incredibly satisfying at the same time—painful, and satisfying, and bizarre . . . And it was only later that I made the connection. What it meant.

And what did it mean?

I had delivered.

Todd started laughing. Which was a good thing because I had to place my hand over the receiver to muffle my own strangling and sputtering noises.

So, did you carry this shared pregnancy through into parenting?
You could say that. It's not completely a fifty-fifty proposition, but it's close. I think I'm more involved than many of the other fathers I know. I cook, I clean, I've changed as many diapers. I do more laundry than Abby does. I do as much of the parenting. I'm just as much their mother as Abby is their father. I love it. I love the nurturing. We even had this problem with the first baby, where she was having a problem with breast-feeding. I got to feed her with a tube and my finger. So she learned to breast-feed on my finger.

So it sounds like you both got there together? Both ended up in the place you wanted to be?
Yes, you could say that. But for all of the experiences we went through together and for all of the things we shared there is something I think that I do resent. I'll never know what it felt like to give birth. She didn't like being pregnant, but she loved giving birth. And I, too, would have loved to feel that. I would give a lot. Physically there was no change and there was a letdown. There was the euphoria of the baby, but I didn't have closure. There was a feeling of anticlimax. We got the baby, yes that's what we wanted. But that's not all I wanted. I wanted me, Todd, to be different.

I wasn't sure quite what to do with all the information Todd had given me. My intuition told me that he had achieved some closure and I wanted to tell him that. Perhaps the largest dump in history was a fitting metaphorical end to his journey? But my thoughts were too half-formed to say anything.

A few days later I was still chuckling when I recalled something from my earlier reading about both creation stories and ritual couvade. After checking some of my references I took another look at a book called *Creation and Procreation: Feminist Reflections on Mythologies of Cosmogony and Parturition*, by Marta Weigle.

Sure enough, after a bit of hunting I found it, a subchapter titled "Defecation and Parturition." It turns out the idea of cloacal birth—godlike figures giving birth to the earth and other cosmic fixtures through their assholes—is a common theme in much of the world's cultural mythologies. What do you make of that? I think that any Freudian worth his or her salt, or for that matter *anyone* who thought about it for thirty seconds would detect some male wish fulfillment here.

OF CALIFORNIA MICE AND MEN

Erica has a subversive streak. At the moment she's gotten all in a tizzy. We've just finished watching videotape of a couple giving birth using the Bradley method. (The Bradley philosophy is very anti–medical establishment and anti-intervention.) I, too, have to admit that the video is hard to take. It was all so . . . unctuous. Mr. and Mrs. Bradley Method are in a birthing room with a midwife. Mrs. BM is laboring away with the requisite concomitant sound effects. Accompanying her moans is a background soundtrack of really awful sitar music emanating out of a boombox the couple has brought to the delivery room. The result sounds like Ravi Shankar trying to play through a heart attack. As Mrs. BM labors, Mr. BM keeps up an unrelenting patter. The dialog between them is some sort of fusion between Harold Pinter and the Marx Brothers.

MR. BM: Let all of the tension leave your body ... visualize your cervix ...

MRS. BM: Oh, it hurts. I hate this. (Swiveling her hips back and forth while squatting on her haunches.)

MR. BM: She feels great.

MRS. BM: Oh, it hurts bad.

MR. BM: It's good that she feels this bad.

MRS. BM: I'm going to black out.

MR. BM: You're on a ship floating up over the waves ...

MRS. BM: How much longer do I have to keep this up?

MR. BM: You're riding down the other side of the wave ... continue to relax to the sound of your breathing ...

MRS. BM: I just want to get this out ...

MR. BM: It's so beautiful at the peak of the wave. The other boats on the water are so pretty. The wave keeps going and floats onto the shore.

MRS. BM: I'm lost.

MR. BM: ... and you're lifting higher and higher on the waves, until you're looking at the stars ...

MRS. BM: I'm out of control.

MR. BM: You're in a nice comfortable position ...

The husband's constant patter is maddening to everyone, including, it seems, to his laboring wife.

MRS. BM (snapping at him): How would you know?

MR. BM (undeterred): Imagine your big bag of muscles contracting, driving the baby toward your cervix ...

After what seems to be an eternity the baby's head starts to crown.

MR. BM: There's going to be a lot of hurt and a lot of burning. It's going to feel like you're going to split . . . but you're not. Okay now, get it out.
MRS. BM: I'm resting, okay?
MR. BM (to the midwife): Can I catch the baby? Can I catch the baby?
MIDWIFE: Yes, yes. Just give me a second.

Finally the baby comes out, but it doesn't start breathing immediately.

MR. BM (to the midwife): He's not breathing. Help him breathe. Help him breathe.

The midwife, flustered, actually slaps the baby twice on its bottom; despite the cliché, it's a no-no these days. It does the trick, however, and the baby starts howling.

MR. BM (to the midwife): Okay, that's enough . . . (cradles the baby) oh, my beautiful little boy . . . what a beautiful little head . . . No, no, I want the blue blanket.

Erica shuts off the tape and turns up the lights. By now the men and women in our class are behaving like the villagers in *Frankenstein*: They're ready to hunt down the monster. "So, what did you think?" Erica asks, sweetly.

The overwhelming consensus: The husband should be killed. Why? "He talked too much . . . he was really over the top . . . he was patronizing . . . controlling . . . hyper . . . selfish . . . he was just absorbed in his mantra, he wasn't really responding to her . . . it was more about his ego than her birth, he wanted to turn it into his experience . . . he tried to define the energy for himself, he totally poisoned it . . . she was in her own world, and he was trying to get in on the action . . ."

The critical mood extended all the way to the baby, who was also criticized for taking too long to cry and breathe.

Finally, Erica weighed in. "What you just watched was the power of belief. No matter what you thought of him or her, what you should consider is that this couple had a plan, they had a script, which they followed. They both walked in there with a belief system and what they believed was supposed to happen, actually did happen.

"So the first question you should ask yourself is, 'Do we actually have a plan?' It's important to have a plan that the both of you have worked out in advance. If you don't have one, what can happen is that both people will retreat inwards.

"The second question you birth partners should ask yourselves is, 'What is it that you expect for yourselves?' It's important for men to feel that they are participating and contributing, but it's also important to expect nothing in return. This goes back to what I said earlier about birth. Birth is not a performance—not for the mother and not for you. In the labor and delivery the emotional energy should be directed at the mother. Many men have a fear of being rejected, some have a fear of not being able to see their partner in pain, and others fear just becoming part of the background.

"The third question is, 'Are you committed to being flexible and to doing what is actually appropriate to the situation?' Sometimes I think that we have been sold a script of what it means to be a labor support person. 'This is what he's supposed to do and when.' These ideas aren't always appropriate. Sometimes just being in the background is enough. Consider when your partner is in pain. You may think that you should be massaging her, but sometimes the woman will say, 'Don't touch me,' and what she really means is, 'This is already enough . . . what I'm going through now in my body is too big to have any more stimulus.' So as partners you have to be flexible. Sometimes things will work out as you planned, sometimes you'll have to make up new rituals spontaneously on the spot.

"One last thing I want birth partners to keep in mind. There are going to be a lot of people involved in the birth process. Most of them are going to be technicians of a sort. All of them have a specific function. You as the birth partner have a different role. Have conviction that part of what you will be doing, just by being there, is keeping the space sacred."

Keeping the space "sacred." It sounded great, but what does it really mean?

Was Erica being nice, or was she being a tad disingenuous? Looking around the room, none of us, women or men, had the faintest idea what we were going to do. We men were especially hopeless. You could see it in our faces, the constantly averted eyes, the middle-distance stares. Maybe Mr. Bradley Method didn't execute perfectly, and maybe he was a bit of a pompous ass, but he had conviction. He believed in what they were doing.

So, what was it about him that made everyone so pissed off? Exasperating as he sounded, he was executing a plan that both of them had agreed on. He was helping her visualize, he was massaging her, and he was actually honest about how much this was going to hurt. All this was more than likely helping her. After all, she wasn't waving him off or cursing him out. So what was the big deal?

The more I think about it, the more I think that this episode explains some of the paradoxes that lie at the heart of this issue. It is particularly instructive that both the men and the women in the class were initially skeptical and disapproving of Mr. BM's behavior. Yet most men and women who go through the birth process barely have belief systems, barely have plans, barely know what's going on, but we'll be damned if we do anything that upsets our image of ourselves. The problem with Mr. BM was that he was behaving, acting, and speaking like a woman. If a woman had been saying or doing those things, everyone would have assumed it was the right thing to do.

When men act within the birth arena, we act without authority and legitimacy. Whose fault is this? Well, it is the fault of men— partly. When it comes to pregnancy, men are petulant and pathetic pioneers. We are constantly playing a game of It, Not It. We pay lip service to being birth partners, but we're uncomfortable with straying into strange territory or behaving in ways that are unfamiliar.

However, there is more than enough blame to go around. We are hardly encouraged by any of the other players in the birth process. Certainly the medical profession doesn't want men assuming a broader role. They are still having trouble digesting the presence of extraneous human variables such as midwives, birth plans, and the desires of mothers. Midwives and the natural birth establishment also deserve their share in the blame. I can remember one midwife bluntly telling me, "This whole business of men being coaches is a lot of bullshit. They should just stay the hell out of the way." The feminist cadres of the birth process, ironically enough, would like to redefine birth as women's work so that they can regain power over it. No wonder men feel uncomfortable. Simply put, the major players and antagonists of the birth process can barely tolerate each other, so they certainly aren't interested in inviting men into the process in a serious way.

Although I disagree with his choice of words and his conclusions, I sympathize with Derek the Hedge Fund Manager's sentiments. Men's participation in pregnancy is, at the moment, perilously close to the level of a sham. It is difficult for men to take themselves seriously because we are not really treated seriously. Lack of seriousness has its consequences. If men don't take the initiative to include themselves, if we are not invited early on into the process, is it any wonder that many men find it difficult to step into the sacred circle of parenting later on?

Where does this confusion of forces leave men? Either passively catatonic or aggressively exploratory, like a mouse in a maze. My own behavior is tending toward the latter. The other day I accompanied Julie to another of her OB/GYN appointments. Dr. Spyros was out, so Dr. Balakian, her partner, was on duty. She was in the middle of performing a cervical exam on Julie when I blurted out, "Can you teach me how to do that?"

"Excuse me?" she said, hesitating and turning toward me with a look that said, "I'm either suffering from auditory hallucinations, or perhaps you are some kind of maniac."

"I was wondering if you could teach me how to do a cervical exam," I continued, swallowing hard. "One of the problems that women have is coming to the hospital too early in the labor. If I could learn how to do a cervical exam, I could make sure that Julie would arrive at the hospital at the right time."

Dr. Balakian gave me a half-smile, half-frown: the smile no doubt relief at not having a neurological episode; the frown, self-explanatory. "I don't think that is a good idea. That's why I pay $100,000 in malpractice insurance every year."

I say nothing in response, but I can't say I agree with her.

After all, I'm not sure that much separates me from the first-year residents who will be performing cervical exams on Julie in the hospital, except for some weeks of study and practice. Maybe my request is a little loopy, but I don't feel that I deserved to be dismissed out of hand. Oh, well, I guess I won't ask her how hard it would be to learn how to do an emergency C-section.

I want to tell her the story of California mice, *Peromyscus californicus*. Genuinely attentive and caring fathers in nature are rare, but there are a few, especially among biparental species. Richard Brown, an animal behaviorist who studies the biparental California mice, discovered that not only are male California mice caring fathers, they also play a big role in the timing of birth, and in the actual delivery itself. Take the male away prior to birth, and the labor is delayed by as much as two days—a long time in mouse gestation. Subsequently, without the male present, the delivery also takes twice as long—fifty-five versus twenty-nine minutes.

During the birth the California mouse male is better than a midwife. The male prepares the female for birth by licking her anogenital region—a form of mouse perineal massage. Throughout the birth the male grooms and licks the female. Then, as each of the two to three pups is born, the male helps by pulling each pup out, licking it off, and getting it settled in the nest.

Finally, when the birthing is over and everything is nice and warm and cozy, the male and the female celebrate by dining together on the placenta.

HOW NATURE MAKES FATHERS OUT OF MEN

My favorite way of responding to potentially life-altering information is asking to hear it again. "Umm . . . Anne, could you say that again, please?"

"I said that we have found that men have a hormonal response to pregnancy which mirrors their partner's hormonal response, and correlates to couvade symptoms," said the small voice on the other end of the line with a somewhat otherworldly timbre.

I was speaking to Anne Storey, in the department of psychology at Memorial University, in St. John's, Newfoundland.* I had been given her number by Bob Elwood—the same Bob Elwood who had written the paper on how couvade syndrome was probably tied to a paternal response. I had called Elwood up on a lark, to talk about his paper, but also to see what he knew beyond what he had already written.

One of the things I found out was how much serendipity and hunches play in science. It turns out that Elwood, normally an expert in the reproductive behaviors of rodents, specifically gerbils, started to think about some of the implications of his work when he had three kids of his own.

"Males should be solicitous of their children and look after them. Even ignoring is a bad thing in evolutionary terms. So in mammalian species, where males are going to be around their young and take care of them, they go through a physiological change into a paternal state. Now I have three children, and certainly with the first one, I never felt any of the couvade syndrome symptoms. But I certainly changed my attitudes toward children during my wife's pregnancy. I began to look at children in supermarkets, which I had never done. So while I don't think that biology should proceed by introspection, that did make me wonder from my biological work."

*A. E. Storey, C. J. Walsh, R. L. Quinton, and K. E. Wynne-Edwards, "Hormonal Correlates of Paternal Responsiveness in New and Expectant Fathers," *Evolution and Human Behavior* (in press).

So these changes don't have to be correlated with couvade syndrome, per se?

I could well imagine that a physiological change could occur and a lot of men wouldn't notice any overt symptoms. I do think that a lot of men notice that they become a lot more solicitous of children, but don't report any problems with their health.

Do you think this behavior is evolutionary?

I think it's adaptive, yes, although feeling sick isn't adaptive. The change is adaptive. The fact that men are becoming more prepared for the arrival of their child, and are prepared to look after them is definitely adaptive.

After I talked with him for about an hour, Elwood passed along Anne Storey's number with what seemed like unbelievable offhandedness. "I told you about Anne Storey who's following up the physiological basis of paternal response in humans. She's a biologist with a variety of interests in animal behavior. She's worked on rodents, but thought that the follow-up on humans was terribly important. I thought about doing humans, but it's not really my field. Besides, I thought that getting the data I wanted would be very difficult. With animals I can arrange pregnancies whenever I want. The idea of tracking down hordes of human males who had just started up relationships with females and hadn't yet started breeding, was mind-boggling."

What Anne Storey did—considering the average human's attitude about having his or her mortal coil unnecessarily punctured—was quietly Herculean. She managed to convince thirty-four expecting couples attending a prenatal class to give blood for her study, leaving one wondering what passes for entertainment in St. John's, Newfoundland. Thirty-one of the couples were expecting their first baby. Couples were tested at three stages: the second trimester; the last three weeks of pregnancy; the first three weeks after their babies were born.

At each stage, two blood tests were taken thirty minutes apart. The first sample was taken shortly after researchers arrived. Then couples were asked to hold a soft-bodied doll wrapped in a receiving blanket that had been worn by a newborn. Then they listened to a tape of newborns crying. Next, they watched a breast-feeding video where a couple greets their newborn and the newborn struggles to nurse for the first time. The idea here was to see if newborn sights, sounds, and smells had an impact on hormone levels. After a half-hour of this, another blood sample was drawn from the expectant mom and dad. Then couples were asked to fill out a questionnaire inquiring about changes in thinking, talking about, and responding to babies, the number and severity of pregnancy symptoms in women and couvade symptoms in men, and the emotional responses of both partners to the tape recording of the baby cries.

This is what she found out.

Men did indeed have a pronounced hormonal response to pregnancy and childbirth, showing significant changes in the three hormones they measured—cortisol, prolactin, and testosterone—from the prenatal to the postnatal period. Cortisol and prolactin levels increased during the prenatal period, peaking at labor and delivery, while testosterone levels dropped significantly immediately after birth.

"I think the strongest finding here is that the cortisol in men tracks the women's cortisol quite nicely," Storey told me over the phone. "Cortisol is normally called a 'stress hormone,' but perhaps a better way of thinking of it is as a hormone that 'alerts' the organism, elevates its awareness of the environment and events. During pregnancy and childbirth, it may help focus attention on the fetus and the newborn and facilitate bonding."

The increase in prolactin in human males is significant because it matches what researchers are finding in other biparental species. Prolactin is an important component in the parental care of birds, and female mammals, and there is evidence that an increase in prolactin in males is an indicator of the onset of paternal care in mammalian species where the father is involved in caring for the young. These include dwarf hamsters, California mice, and tamarin monkeys.

The fall-off in testosterone in human males after the birth of the baby is interesting because again it matches patterns found in other biparental species. For example, in ring doves (most birds are biparental), testosterone peaks in early courtship and declines afterward, followed by an increase in prolactin during incubation and brooding. As Storey cites so delicately in her paper, "the high levels of testosterone during the courtship and mating phases must decrease in order for males to engage in competent parental behavior, primarily because testosterone enhances the frequency of non-parental activities."

What all this suggests is that expectant human fathers, like many other species, undergo physiological changes during the pregnancy period that sensitize and prime them for parenthood. Furthermore, some men have a stronger response than others.

"Men with couvade syndrome, for our purposes those with two or more symptoms, had a more intense response to the baby cries in the test, and both they and their partners had higher levels of prolactin," said Storey. "Another thing that is interesting is that while men with more symptoms reported more anxiety, they also reported higher levels of happiness. So it seems possible that increased cortisol is part of a general increase in emotional responsiveness during this period."

What do you think triggers this change? Men and women living together?

It's hard to say at this point. No one has been able to pin it down, even in animal studies. In different species it's different social cues, like it could be the arrival of the young themselves that kick off these changes. But in humans these changes are happening before the babies are born. So you get a situation where males would be more likely to be involved when the babies are born.

I think the correlation between male cortisol and female hormone levels suggests an interesting factor for further study. Changes in male cortisol may occur as a response to partners' changes in hormones. A similar synchronization of hormones has been shown in courting monogamous birds, such as the ring dove.

So you're talking about synchronization going on between expectant mothers and fathers?

That's probably what is going on here, the pregnant partner getting the other one up to speed, but maybe I can't say that yet. In ring doves the crop milk that both parents secrete to feed the babies is all prolactin induced. It starts with the initial mating. He sees her. His testosterone level goes up. Her estradiol goes up. They go through the mating, picking the nest site, the nest-build . . . then they start to incubate. Their steroids drop to near nothing, while their prolactin goes up as they incubate. But they need each other to start doing it. They are synchronizing each other, pacing each other.

Those doves ring a bell. Sounds oddly familiar.
Anyway, that's the bird perspective.

THAT EXPLAINS EVERYTHING

You will reply that reality hasn't the slightest need to be of interest. And I'll answer you that reality may avoid the obligation to be interesting, but that hypotheses may not. In the hypothesis you have postulated, chance intervenes largely.

—Jorge Luis Borges, *Death and the Compass*

Synchronizing each other . . .

Can some of the wacky behavior that women and men go through during pregnancy be explained by hormones? Is there a paternal response as well as a maternal response?

First, let's take a look at the maternal response. Between the hormonally influenced reproductive and parental behavior of lower mammals and modern women talking about their pregnancy is an evolutionary story that spans millions of years and, I believe, explains something about who we are today. Quoting David Crews, an evolutionary biologist from the University of Texas, "it long has been recognized that behavior is the leading edge of evolutionary change, but only recently has it been realized that reproductive behaviors, in particular, have a 'disproportionate influence on brain evolution.'"*

*D. Crews, "Evolutionary Antecedents to Love," *Psychoneuroendocrinology* 23, no. 8 (1998), p. 756.

The changes that take place in the Kate Spade diaper bag–buying, Baby Gap–obsessed, pregnancy tome–reading, cracker-chewing, can't-stop-talking-to-my-friends pregnant woman are a marvel of evolutionary engineering. But given the amount of investment that mammalian young require, a lot more is required for reproductive success from mothers than merely the physical act of giving birth. What is required is a certain set of reliable nurturing behaviors; and so, more revealing and remarkable is the fact that various hormones driving the physical changes of pregnancy also, in many cases, act as neurotransmitters, connecting the endocrine system with structures and systems in the brain that are central to sexual and social behavior. Binding all this together is the hypothalamus, a master control organ that not only orchestrates reproduction, but also connects to the limbic system, a series of ancient mid-brain structures (many of which are common to all vertebrates), basic to our emotions, motivation, memory, and learning. Finally, the limbic system interacts with our cortex, or the most evolved part of our brain, which controls, among many things, language.

So what we are talking about here is the idea that pregnancy is much more than a "physical" process. The hormones of pregnancy that trigger and regulate body changes also simultaneously trigger and regulate changes in our behavior. This makes perfect sense. A body ramping up to give birth to and nurture life with everything from nutrients, immune agents, and physical protection and comfort should be acting in concert with a mind also preparing for motherhood by increasing its emotional commitment, focusing its attention, and enhancing its cognitive faculties. In short, a pregnant body should have a pregnant mind.

PREGNANT MIND

One major feature of the pregnant brain is that it is driving a dramatic and permanent change in behaviors. The pregnant mind is in transition, *becoming* a maternal mind, just as a pregnant woman is in the process of becoming a mother. As Bob Elwood said in his conversation with me, "Being female is not the same thing as being maternal. It has to be triggered by some mechanism." This shift in behavior, called a maternal response, is the essence of all mammalian motherhood, whether you live in a large ugly Tudor in Scarsdale or in a burrow. This maternal bond is in turn part of a larger dynamic of social behaviors that scientists call affiliative or attachment behaviors, which form the basis of our families and our societies. These bonds also include the pair-bond between male and female sexual partners, and, it would appear now, the bond between father and child. Many of these behaviors seem to be influenced by hormones.

How does the maternal response work? What would have turned the callow Paleolithic teenager who cared only about showing off her beadwork into a mother? The short answer to the question is that the brain actually has to change structurally. The exact mechanism of maternal response is more mystery than knowledge at this point, but scientists have begun identifying what appear to be some of the major hormonal, genetic, and neural systems and subsystems.

Estrogen and progesterone seem to be the chief architect and master builder of the maternal response. The idea that a sex steroid, estrogen, gets the behavioral ball rolling makes a lot of sense when you think of the effect that sex steroids have in all the major biological transitions of our lives, not to mention whether we become "male" or "female." The release of estrogen at the beginning of pregnancy initiates and orchestrates a cascade of events. It interacts with the individual's genome, switching on genes that are specifically related to maternal behavior and processes, as well as activating the release and enabling the effects of other hormones.

From the very beginning the pregnant mind is in a state of dynamic change. It becomes "plastic," meaning it is malleable and capable of being re-formed. Estrogen controls this process by actually "growing," shaping, and improving the communicative capacities of certain brain pathways. Think of it as a computer network that receives increased memory and faster pipelines, along with a new program that redirects resources toward specific, pregnancy-related goals. Recent studies on mice by Craig Kinsley at the University of Richmond show that the higher hormone levels of pregnancy double the density of dendrites and glial cells in the hippocampus, a part of the brain's limbic system involved in memory. The result of all this construction? Mice mothers who were bolder, more curious and energetic, learned mazes more quickly, made fewer mistakes, and retained new information longer than other mice.*

Estrogen facilitates other hormones, most notably prolactin, a pituitary hormone that scientists believe is another key player in maternal response. The action of these hormones seems to converge on an area of the brain called the medial preoptic area (MPOA) of the basal forebrain, a staging area for maternal mechanisms. The MPOA seems to be an interface between the

---

*C. H. Kinsley, E. A. Amory, J. Wartella, G. W. Gifford, and K. G. Lambert, "Pregnancy Drives Modifications in Neurogenesis and Hippocampal Neural and Glial Morphology and Activity," presented at the Maternal Brain Conference, University of Bristol, July 1999.

endocrine system and the key behavioral structures of the brain, receiving input from and outputting to areas of the limbic system that are involved in emotions, memory, and motivation.*

Another key feature of the pregnant brain is its reaction and relationship to stress. Predating Anne Storey's findings, Alison Fleming of the University of Toronto—one of the foremost researchers in maternal response, and one of the few who has actually conducted extensive human studies—has found that high levels of cortisol during pregnancy are the best predictor of the intensity and quality of maternal attachment after the child is born.† Cortisol may also act as a staging hormone for other mechanisms. One possibility pointed out by Sue Carter of the University of Maryland is that high levels of cortisol may enable the behavioral effects of oxytocin and vasopressin, two very similar hormones that have been implicated in maternal behavior. Oxytocin is released during childbirth and lactation and has been correlated during breast-feeding with feelings of calmness, increased sociability, and a willingness to please. Vasopressin has been implicated in pair bonding in male prairie voles, a biparental species, and is linked to territoriality and guarding behavior, as well as obsessive behaviors.‡

The brain changes, the mind changes, behavior changes. Being female is not the same thing as being maternal, but what is it that exactly defines becoming maternal? This may sound obvious but

*M. Numan, "Maternal Behavior," in *The Physiology of Reproduction*, edited by E. Knobil and J. D. Neill (Raven Press, 1994), p. 263.

†A. S. Fleming, M. Steiner, and C. Corter, "Cortisol, Hedonics, and Maternal Responsiveness in Human Mothers," *Hormones and Behavior* 32 (1997): pp. 85–98.

‡C. S. Carter, "Neuroendocrine Perspectives on Social Attachment and Love," *Psychoneuroendocrinology* 23, no. 8 (1998): pp. 779–818.

it's important to realize that a woman who is pregnant cares about different things, acts on different thoughts, and relates to herself and others in different ways than when she wasn't pregnant. In dynamic relationship with brain systems, hormones influence our mental state, our mood, and our disposition toward one thing over another, and thus ultimately how we act. This changing "phenomenology" of a pregnant woman's mind—the way her brain perceives, orders, ranks, prioritizes, and gives meaning to information—is perhaps the most salient feature of pregnancy. Male partners complain and sulk about being "abandoned" because they are on the receiving end of this change in priorities. The male ego tends to misinterpret this change as a loss of importance, but what are you going to do? The pregnant woman's pregnant mind is shifting its priorities and resources.

What drives these changes? You have to be careful to distinguish between pregnancy *attitudes* and pregnancy *behaviors*, as Alison Fleming pointed out to me. Women can be quite ambivalent about being pregnant for all sorts of reasons—doubts about becoming a parent, doubts about the father, growing physical discomfort, and so on—but their behaviors tend to progress toward preparation and growing emotional attachment.

Paradoxes abound in pregnancy because pregnancy behaviors are driven by what I think of as the seemingly paradoxical relationship between the mechanisms that drive the mammalian stress response and the mechanisms that protect against psychological and physical stress. I mean, why aren't pregnant women lunatics? They have to endure long periods of intense and acute physical and psychological stress. They also have to endure the knowledge—since humans are also self-aware beings—that their bodies are changing radically. Why don't these forces combine to create pregnant women who are crazed?

The answer is, pregnant woman are bomb-proof. Yes, pregnant women can be seemingly "out of it," absent-minded and forgetful, at times irritable, obsessional, and overemotional, but what is truly remarkable is how well pregnant women function. An amazing study on women who had been pregnant during the California earthquake of 1994 showed that women actually decreased their psychological response to acute stress as their pregnancy progressed. Women who had been in their third trimester when the quake struck barely registered concern at all.*

How can this be? It seems so counter-intuitive; one would expect pregnant women to be more anxious.

BRAIN CANDY

The answer is that the pregnant woman's brain is flooded with "brain candy." Estrogen, prolactin, and progesterone are involved in activating neural systems essential to mood and motivation and cranking them up to the setting marked "high." Estrogen and prolactin are both involved in modulating systems, such as the GABA (gamma-aminobutyric acid) system of inhibitory neurotransmitters that are responsible for turning brain synapses off (GABA receptors are those acted upon by benzodiazepam, read Valium); the dopamine system, (read cocaine); the serotonin system, (read Prozac); the endogenous opioid system, such as endorphins (read heroin); and the norepinephrine system, which is important to arousal and selective attention. And these are just the systems that scientists have been able to isolate up to now. There are undoubt-

*L. M. Glynn, P. D. Wadhwa, D. Dunkel-Schetter, and C. A. Sandman, "Pregnancy Decreases Psychological Response to Acute Stress," paper presented at the Maternal Brain Conference, University of Bristol, July 1999.

edly more involved. So powerful are these mechanisms that schizophrenic women who suffer from acute episodes when pregnant are usually able to weather them without breaking down. Personally speaking, this brain candy is the big reason that Julie has so far sailed through the pregnancy without her Wellbutrin. She constantly remarks about how good she feels, even better than when she is taking her antidepressant medication. Amen.

All this brain candy creates what I call the "pregnancy head." Anxiety, which is a big part of pregnancy, should be thought of in a more complex way than just nervousness or apprehension. Expectant mothers definitely need to have a stress response—cortisol, as Anne Storey suggests, "alerts the organism to events that are happening in the environment." The high levels of cortisol in the system raises the "salience" of anything pregnancy-related, enhancing a pregnant woman's responses to her environment, and the people in it. Consequently, it changes what the mind is aware of, attributes meaning to, and chooses to act upon.

The brain candy is what keeps the stress response positive, constructive, and bearable. I think it's the anxiety-reducing effect of dopamine, opioids, serotonin, and the GABA system that dampens the negative effects of the high levels of cortisol, leaving the sensory acuity, heightened environmental sensitivity, and selective arousal. The result is a combination of hyperawareness, a sense of urgency without anxiety, extreme selectivity, an ability to learn at a remarkable rate, and single-mindedness that pregnant women exhibit especially late in pregnancy when they start "nesting."

How does all this add up to increasing attachment and a maternal response? How does all this add up to love? Let's begin by thinking about it in the reverse. How can mothers gaze upon newborns with such intense joy and love immediately after going through the most painful experience of their lives? Weird, no?

Think of what's required to not kill your kid after a month of colicky sleep deprivation. It's no wonder that God is a pharmacist. You don't even have to have been a heavy drug user to understand that these buffering systems might be crucial to attachment and affiliation, especially when they interact dynamically with the brain's emotional and motivational limbic interface.

WHOSE BRAIN, WHOSE CANDY?

The question is, who benefits the most from all of this dramatic and radical physiological change in the mother? The answer that turns everything on its head is that most of these changes are to the advantage of the fetus, not the mother. Furthermore, what we think of as mother love and maternal attachment is not wholly a function of the mother's physiology. In fact, the whole phenomenon of pregnancy—certainly the maternal physiology, and perhaps the maternal state of mind—is the result of a dialog of common and conflicting interests between mother and fetus.

While the mother and fetus share the same end goal—which is a successful delivery—the amount of maternal resources allocated to the pregnancy is a matter of contention. Harvard zoologist David Haig has argued that much of the hormonal phenomena of pregnancy is the result of an "arms race" of adaptations that have emerged over evolutionary time, enabling the mother and fetus to negotiate the physiological conditions of pregnancy.* Fetal involvement begins with implantation, when the fetus invades the lining of the uterus, forms the placenta, and gains access to the

*David Haig, "Genetic Conflicts in Human Pregnancy," *Quarterly Review of Biology* 68 (1993): pp. 485–532.

mother's bloodstream. By releasing its hormones through this "maternal-fetal interface" into the maternal bloodstream, the fetus gains influence over maternal organs and regulatory systems.

The placenta becomes, essentially, another endocrine organ in the mother's body. Placental HCG (human chorionic gonadotrophin) stimulates the release of more progesterone, which helps protect the fetus against miscarriage. Placental lactogens raise the mother's blood sugar levels to provide more nutrients. The fetus also acts to raise the mother's blood pressure so that more blood is pumped into the placenta. (Imbalances in these last two conditions can lead to pregnancy-induced diabetes and pre-eclampsia.)

Haig's description of the fetus's interaction with the mother's physiology provides a basis for speculating about the fetus's influence over the maternal mind. Certainly this is what happens in other mammals. As Robert Bridges of Tufts has shown in rats, the release of placental lactogens helps to prime the pregnant female rat's brain to respond maternally at the end of gestation.[*] In human mothers, the phenomenon of "pregnancy head" that I described—a constructive stress response of elevated anxiety mediated with anti-anxiety agents—could be due partially to the fetus's influence. Progesterone is metabolized into a neurosteroid that stimulates the GABA system, or the brain's "valium."[†] The release of placental CRF or (corticotropin-releasing factor) could have a direct effect on the mother's HPA (hypothalamic-pituitary-adrenal) axis, resulting in the regulation of cortisol production in the mother's adrenal glands.[‡]

[*]R. S. Bridges, "The Role of Lactogenic Hormones in Maternal Behavior in Female Rats," *Acta Paediatrica*, suppl. 397 (1994), pp. 33–39.

[†]Thomas Insel, personal communication.

[‡]Alison Fleming, personal communication.

Maternal HPA activity correlates with the quality of maternal response. Alison Fleming correlated higher levels of cortisol during pregnancy with a higher quality of maternal response to infants postpartum. The fetal influence on maternal response makes adaptive sense. In humans where the amount of maternal investment necessary is so enormous, it is to the fetus's advantage to get an early start in making sure the mother is prepared for motherhood.

For the fetus, it would be an advantage to have a mother buffered from physiological and psychological stress so she can concentrate on the preparations for birth. It would be an advantage to have a mother whose elevated brain chemistry is making her resilient, acutely aware, selective, goal-directed, and self-transcendent. It would be an advantage to have a mother who is more social, seeking out support from relatives, other women, and most of all, the father—generally making sure that all of the relationships that will carry her and her fetus through pregnancy, birth, and parenting, are strong and in place.

So, are men also programmed by nature to be paternal?

The idea of a maternal response seems obvious and universal. But a paternal response? To many women, especially those who have just witnessed their husbands heading out the door to the golf course, it seems counterintuitive. (Nature would support women in this view. More than 90 percent of mammalian species are non-paternal.) Men have a wide-ranging response to their own children both within cultures and across cultures. Sure, there are a few men who care for children as much as their wives, and a larger number who cooperate in child care, but there are plenty of others who rarely seem to pay attention to their children at all. How could there be a paternal response?

Actually, the real issue is not whether men are paternal. Human males—unlike the vast majority of male mammals—are extremely paternal. All hunter-gatherer fathers invest huge amounts of time and energy in the care of their children. What confuses us moderns is that the care males invest is rarely hands-on care. (In preindustrial societies, infants are always attached to the mother because they need constant access to the breast.) Paternal investment usually comes in the form of providing food, protection, shelter, and teaching. It also may take the form of the passing on of the father's status through the acknowledgment of paternity, a form of investment that should not be underestimated. A father acknowledging paternity can make the difference between life and death, as well as bestow future psychological well-being on the child.

The real issues are: Is this paternal care and investment driven by some physiological process? How would it work physiologically? What were the forces that created and shaped it evolutionarily? And what do these forces reveal about the nature of reproduction, parenting, and human nature in general?

To reveal my bias, I think the circumstantial evidence for a physiological paternal response is considerable and compelling. Most fathers I have spoken to—including among them many biologists—state emphatically that their feelings and behavior are different after the birth of a child. They are more emotional. They are more caring. They take fewer risks. And they are more interested in not only their own children, but also children in general. Men have pregnancy symptoms in large numbers. Many men have strong and intense reactions to their newborns, a phenomenon that has been tagged with the unfortunate name of "engrossment." Psychologists have noted and catalogued the "pregnancy careers" of men.

Certainly, the quantifiable predictability of much of men's

behavioral changes suggests that there is a process at work. More importantly, when you factor in the absolutely crucial importance of paternal cooperation and investment in the face of encephalization and the environmental challenges facing ancestral humans, there are plenty of reasons to think that many evolutionary adaptations are essentially paternal adaptations. The behavior is too important to leave to learning or chance. As David Gubernick of UC Davis puts it, "animals could not evolve ... long-term, reciprocal, mutualistic, intimate relationships ... with non-kin without also evolving mechanisms to ensure that, on average, each member of the cooperating unit received reproductive benefits greater than he or she would receive if acting alone or in cooperating with others."[*]

But is there proof that human males are primed hormonally for fatherhood? Anne Storey's findings are not absolute proof of a biologically based, paternal response but it certainly makes the circumstantial case extremely suggestive and powerful. The critical findings in her study to focus on are: (1) Men in general had a hormonal response to pregnancy that "mapped" their partner's response, that is, elevated levels of cortisol and prolactin during pregnancy with a drop in testosterone following birth.[†] (2) This type of response is identical to the hormonal response in males of mammal species that are biparental, and notable for its absence in species that are not biparental. (3) One of the strongest and most significant correla-

[*]Gubernick, "Biparental Care and Male-Female Relations in Mammals," in S. Parmigiani and F. S. von Saal, eds., *Infanticide and Parental Care* (Chur, Switzerland: Harwood Academic Publishers, 1994), pp. 427–63.

[†]Also supporting her work are earlier findings by Gubernick, who reported a drop in testosterone in men following the birth of a child. D. J. Gubernick, C. M. Worthman, and J. F. Stallings, "Hormonal Correlates of Fatherhood in Men," paper presented at the meeting of the International Society of Developmental Psychobiology, October 1992.

tions was that variations in hormonal response and concern for infants were correlated to the strength of pregnancy symptoms in both females *and* males. She also found that men with couvade— which she defined as two or more pregnancy symptoms—had a greater degree of measurable hormonal responsiveness. The idea that this in turn is correlated to paternal response is further supported by other studies that correlate strength of couvade symptoms to a higher quality of infant care postpartum.

The idea that couvade syndrome is strongly correlated to paternal response is extremely suggestive because if the data on couvade syndrome is at all reliable, it could indicate that paternal response might be a nearly universal phenomenon. As I discussed earlier, couvade syndrome has been documented in countries around the world, including the United States, Canada, Britain, Scandinavia, Italy, and Thailand. While the incidence varies widely in these studies, from about 20 percent to over 90 percent, as I said before, one of the most conservative of studies, by Mack Lipkin of NYU— where men actually had to complain of their symptoms to a health care practitioner—recorded an incidence rate of nearly a quarter of the men in the study, indicating that the actual rate of couvade symptoms was probably much higher.

Anne Storey and Catherine Courage conducted a recent couvade syndrome survey that reported over 90 percent of men reported more than two pregnancy-related symptoms.* What explains the great difference in results? A variety of factors come into play. Ways of soliciting and measuring responses differ. Cultural attitudes differ. Perhaps the strongest reason: Older studies took place in a milieu where symptoms would have been stigma-

---

*C. Courage, "Couvade Syndrome: A Biological Perspective," honors thesis, Department of Psychology, Memorial University of Newfoundland, May 1997.

tizing, thus inhibiting men from reporting symptoms. Today, presented in the light that symptoms may actually represent a positive involvement in pregnancy, more men may take notice and come forward. Depending on your inclinations, you could either insist that the data were inconclusive, or you could also make an argument that couvade syndrome is actually a marker for the most overt form of what could be a universal paternal response.

How might this mechanism work in a man's brain? The only model we have at the moment are California mice. David Gubernick has found that neural circuitry underlying paternal behavior is already present in virgin males and he has speculated that a paternal response may require an activation of the neurons in these circuits.* This circuitry, found in the medial preoptic area (MPOA) of the limbic system is inhibited or shielded in virgin males by testosterone. After mating, and just before the birth of young, testosterone levels drop with the result that circulating maternal hormones, such as estrogen and progesterone can then act on the MPOA. (Gubernick's estrogen theory is also supported by the work of Jay Rosenblatt of Rutgers University, who induced "maternal" behavior in rat males by implanting estrogen into the MPOA.)† Since the MPOA is potentially the interface between the endocrine system and the limbic system, a change in its neuronal activity would then indicate a source for a change in emotional responsiveness and behavior.

This also seems to be a common adaptation across a range of other mammalian species that are biparental and monogamous,

---

*D. J. Gubernick, D. R. Sengelaub, and E. M. Kurz,, "A Neuroanatomical Correlate of Paternal and Maternal Behavior in the Biparental California Mouse," *Behavioral Neuroscience*, 107, no. 1 (1993): 194–201.

†J. S. Rosenblatt, personal communication.

such as tamarins, Mongolian hamsters, and prairie voles. They of all of mammals bear the most resemblance to humans in their reproductive strategies, and they all have a paternal priming mechanism, which changes the emotional responsiveness of males toward offspring, most involving an elevation in cortisol and prolactin, and a drop in testosterone.

How would this paternal response be linked physiologically to couvade symptoms? Elwood and Mason suggested that "the couvade syndrome in male humans is better explained as being due to physiological changes that mediate paternal responsiveness. That is, the various psychosomatic symptoms that constitute the couvade syndrome are a perception and interpretation of the normal processes in the male that bring about parental responsiveness." I would guess that the ability to express couvade symptoms and paternal response behavior arise from the same source: the priming of the mechanisms that drive affiliation and bonding. These emotional mechanisms are already in place as part of larger system of empathy and identification that humans use in relationships.

The adaptive value of a paternal response in males is a natural when you consider what it takes to raise human children. It makes sense to have a mechanism that helps men bond with and invest in their children, and conversely, it also makes sense to have a mechanism that ensures that a father doesn't harm his own children. The question that remains is, do couvade symptoms have any function or utility on their own that may be adaptive, or are they, as Elwood and Mason argue, merely a by-product of the underlying physiological changes of a paternal response? Adaptive behaviors result from some pressure that makes them a particularly good solution to social and/or environmental problem, creating a reproductive advantage. What could be reproductively advantageous about throwing up with your wife? I called up Donald

Symons—author of *The Evolution of Human Sexuality** and one of the founders of the field of evolutionary psychology—to see if he could help me sort it all out.

"It's always important to consider the costs," he said. "In this case if you're proposing that husbands of pregnant women evolved to experience pregnancy sickness, and to be lassitudinous when their wives were due, that's not adaptive behavior. That's maladaptive behavior. It's a serious cost. In fact, instead of this type of behavior being passed on genetically, you would expect it to be weeded out over evolutionary time.

"So if you're going to propose that it's adaptive, there's got to be a strong compensatory benefit. You also have to ask yourself, 'What is the functional link between a man feeling nauseous in his partner's first trimester, and that man getting meat or changing diapers after the baby is born?'

"The thing that pops into my mind is 'honest signaling.' Signaling to the mate that you are going to invest. I think this kind of thing goes on not just with couvade; I think it can be placed in the larger context of interpersonal signaling in general. I mean if your mate cries because of something that happened to her and you cry, too, that's telling her something. It's a signal of your feelings about her. In general human communication is full of 'honest signaling.' Why is it that we can read each other's emotions accurately? It's not automatically apparent why something that's going on internally needs to be manifested externally. There are billions of things going on in our bodies that are not manifested on the surface. The fact that emotions are manifested that way, I think tells us something about our ancestral situation. We

*New York: Oxford University Press, 1979.

evolved in small face-to-face kin groups where honest advertising of emotions and the ability to read emotions was adaptive. I'm wondering if couvade is the same thing."

Why do you think it would have been so important for the man to signal to his wife during pregnancy?

In any social relations, whenever you have two roles that come together for any purpose, where the interests are not 100 percent identical—as it is almost all of the time—you have the extreme likelihood of an evolutionary arms race. Clearly that has to be the case in male-female relations. Both have an interest in the child; if the child doesn't survive then it hurts both their interests. But it's very unlikely that all of their interests are identical. It's in the interest of the mother to have as much of the father's investment as possible going into the child. That may not be the male's interest. The male's interest may be to have something less than that. Maybe it's 95 percent into the child and five percent on the side with someone else.

Accordingly, females may have evolved to constantly assess the male's investment reliability. Females have always faced the problem of desertion, or at least lowered invest-ment by males. Late stages of pregnancy are often times when males find other lovers. A pregnant woman is in a very risky situation. She's committed now to this pregnancy, to this enormous investment of time and energy and a situation where it's extremely important to have paternal investment after birth. One of the things that females are selected to do is monitor their mates closely to pick up signs of whether this investment will or will not be forthcoming. It certainly would not surprise me that couvade is a form of male advertising

about paternal commitment. It's a signal about your invest-ment in your mate and in your future offspring. Feeling nau-seous is an honest signal because it's a costly signal. Cost tends to be a guarantee of honesty.

But how does this play out? The man signals his intentions, the wife has more confidence—how does this add up to an advan-tage? The wife is already pregnant.

After birth she still has a choice. She can kill the infant. She has a choice in the degree and quality of the care that she gives the children. As Edward Hagen has demostrated, she can expe-rience postpartum depression, threatening the father with defection from the child. Her investment even extends to the pregnancy period itself. Is she going to take care of herself? Is she going to make sure that the fetus is not injured in any way?

We finished up our conversation on the topic of variation. "Variation gives you something to work with. Couvade could be what we call a *facultative* adaptation, a behavior which occurs in some circumstances and not in others. Everybody has the ability to tan, but you only tan with exposure to the sun. Couvade might have certain specific circumstances that trigger it, and if so, it would be very interesting to know what they are. Who gets it and who doesn't? Is there a systematic variation? Do we have to pro-pose that couvade in particular is an adaptation? I would be interested in knowing if you compared men who had pregnancy symptoms with those who don't, did the men who experienced couvade tend to experience more of their wives' moods in gen-eral? Which would have nothing to do with pregnancy. If their wives are moody, are they moody? Clearly we are evolved to expe-rience things based on our perceptions of other people's feelings.

You're suggesting that couvade be part of a larger way of identifying between men and women?

What I am proposing is that it may not be an adaptation at all. It may just be a manifestation of a more general adaptive tendency to identify with people that we are very close to, but if I were going to explore this as an adaptation I would concentrate on finding a signal. Presumably it would be a signal to one's mate that I'm invested in this child. I care about this child. I recognize it as being my child. I'm going to invest in this child. It would be interesting to know if men who have suspicions about paternity would be less likely to experience couvade.

It would also be interesting to know whether the male's symptoms parallel those of his wife. Do women who tend to experience pregnancy sickness tend to have husbands who have pregnancy sickness? Do women who don't have symptoms have husbands who express the couvade in some other way? In other words, does the husband's experience of pregnancy track his wife's experience of pregnancy?

I'll bet it does. If you say that women have quite different experiences of pregnancy, I'll bet it turns out that the husband's experience of couvade tracks those variations. It would trigger not a specific set of symptoms but a "rule" that you would monitor your wife and express a set of symptoms that are parallel to hers. If so, it would somewhat support the notion that there is communication going on.

So is couvade syndrome a sort of natural Empathy Belly?

I came away from my conversation with Symons with the understanding that the social arrangement we think of as the "family" is shaped as much by conflicts of interest as mutual goals. As Symons put it at one point, "one of the primary sources of the conflict is the amount of investment each parent makes in the offspring. It's not a question of do fathers contribute, or do they contribute 'a lot'; it's a question of whether the optimal paternal investment from the father's point of view is identical to his optimal investment from the mother's point of view. Usually what happens is that fathers are attempting to invest what is optimal for their lifetime reproductive success, and mothers are attempting to obtain more investment than that. This battle does not end with marriage or pregnancy or childbirth; it never ends because, in evolutionary perspective, there is never a perfect overlap of interests. It's this kind of perspective that will make clear the possibility of couvade symptoms as adaptation."

In general, the conflicting interests of the parents make the existence of a communication system not only plausible, but important. If both sides had perfectly aligned interests, no communication would be necessary. The idea that symptoms would be the medium of this signaling also makes sense. Why? Because symptoms are not merely by-products of physiological processes, but external manifestations of internal states, both physiological and emotional, making this type of information important to both parties.

To argue that symptoms, both male and female, are meaningless by-products is calling nature a sloppy designer. When you consider that selection engineered a human eye with rods in it that can detect one photon of light, this is a hard claim to make, especially so when you consider that symptoms carry a substantial cost.* Throwing up means losing a meal's worth of calories. Feeling depressed and otherwise lassitudinous means

*Donald Symons, personal communication.

losing valuable foraging or hunting time. Similarly, nausea and vomiting in women are not "byproducts" of the general physiological changes of pregnancy. As Margie Profet of the University of Washington has convincingly argued, they are the result of specific adaptations that protect the fetus from harmful toxins during the first trimester of development.*

Adaptations arose for specific reasons, engineered by selection in response to specific pressures in the environment. If couvade symptoms are indeed a signaling system, its adaptive value would depend upon whether or not it solves a key social or environmental problem that has an effect on reproductive success, that is, whether or not one's child makes it to reproductive age. What is this key problem? I think it is whether the mother, as well as the father, will choose to invest in the child when it is born.

This is controversial territory. Everyone agrees that women need to perceive men's real intentions and predict their behavior, and men need to make convincing promises. However, while some evolutionary psychologists stress the idea, as Symons did, that mothers need to assess the parenting investment of the father throughout the reproductive cycle, many biologists assume that the only really effective female decision-making point comes with the decision to mate. Once the woman is pregnant, they contend, there is very little a woman can do to counter negative male behavior. What good is monitoring and promises, they say, if mothers can't take some corrective action? Any argument for couvade as a signaling system would need to be supported by evidence showing that decision-making about parental investment for women

---

*M. Profet, 1992. "Pregnancy Sickness as Adaptation: A Deterrent to Maternal Ingestion of Teratogens," in J. Barkow, L. Cosmides, and J. Tooby, eds., *The Adapted Mind* (New York: Oxford University Press, 1992), pp. 327–365.

extends beyond mating, and that women have adaptations that would allow them to respond to lowered investment on the part of the male.

Certainly one response is that most hunter/gatherers practice infanticide. (Frankly, infanticide seems rather common in modern societies also.) As Symons notes in his *The Evolution of Human Sexuality*, a "common problem (among hunter/gatherers) is the birth of infants who cannot be reared; a hunter/gather woman cannot rear more than one child every third or fourth year, and all known aboriginal hunter/gatherer groups practice systematic infanticide."* In such an environment—low birth rate, high infant mortality, high investment threshold—men's behavior has a direct effect on whether or not the mother invests in the child, and selection among men to reliably signal parental intention would be beneficial.

Infanticide, however, is definitely a last resort, since it has drastic consequences for both parents. One would expect other adaptations to emerge which would negotiate a better outcome. Edward Hagen's work on postpartum depression addresses exactly this point, and casts considerable light on the parental investment decision-making process and its adaptations.† Hagen, an evolutionary psychologist at the University of California, Santa Barbara, has shown that postpartum depression has little or nothing to do with the hormonal situation postpartum, and instead is most strongly correlated to the support of the father. In situations where the father is showing little support, Hagen hypothesizes that postpartum depression is a way the mother can threaten him with

*D. Symons, *The Evolution of Human Sexuality* (New York: Oxford University Press, 1979), p. 122.

†E. H. Hagen, "The Functions of Postpartum Depression," *Evolution and Human Behavior* (in press).

defection from the child and thus negotiate an increase in his investment, or if that investment is not forthcoming, depression is a prelude to killing or abandoning the child herself.

Hagen's work gives us at least three important principles to illuminate couvade. First, the response of the father has a direct physiological effect on the health of the mother and the quality of her maternal care. Second, parental investment is not automatic even for a mother. A truer picture of the nature of parental investment is that each parent's investment is contingent on the other, and that both parent's are involved in negotiating levels of parental investment. Third, the process of assessing a mate's parental reliability and then taking some action that has reproductive consequences extends beyond mating to include pregnancy and the postpartum period.

This last point is crucial. As Hagen says, "There is a pervasive bias among biologists that the big decision for females is whether to mate or not. For many mammals that may be the case, but for humans the amount of investment postpartum is enormous. You may be investing in this offspring for the next fifteen or twenty years. It's massive. If you're going to pay a very high price to nurse an infant and raise it to adulthood, the real decision point is not whether to mate but whether to invest postpartum. The sooner you can make that determination the better. The first year postpartum is going to be a time of intense scrutiny and evaluation of the quality of the infant and the nature of the social environment, including the amount of investment from the father."[*]

Once you accept the idea that the most critical moment in decision-making is not the decision to mate but the decision postpartum to invest and raise a child, a much broader range of

[*]Hagen, personal communication.

behavior, including pregnancy behavior, begins to make sense, especially when you consider that much of it involves a tension between conflicting interests and adaptations. In such an environment couvade symptoms would be adaptive for the role they would play in enabling a reliable exchange of information about future parenting intentions and ability.

Given what we know, how might such a system of adaptations, including signaling between partners, work? Starting with Anne Storey's ideas, the female "signals" the male through a physiological mechanism that takes place during co-habitation, in an attempt to trigger the male's paternal response and synchronize it with her own. (Perhaps one reason for the acute awareness of mothers during pregnancy, is that men are possibly adapted to seek other opportunities during this time, when partners are less able physically to keep tabs on them.) Triggering the male's paternal response results in priming affiliative mechanisms also involved in couvade symptoms. Couvade symptoms, then, would be one way that the female could assess the male's paternal response. His level of emotionality, the degree of his identification with the mother, his disposition toward the fetus, his preparations for fatherhood, all might provide a set of criteria to predict his behavior once the child is born.

Given what's at stake, the male, as Symons brought up, would be adapted to follow a "rule" to monitor the mother's physical and emotional state, and then express a set of symptoms that would communicate empathy, identification, and intention. Signaling the female would definitely be adaptive for the male because his expression of support would have a direct effect on the female's attitude toward the pregnancy and toward the baby postpartum. Essentially, the quality of the male's response to the pregnancy helps determine the quality of the female's response.

From an evolutionary viewpoint, pregnancy is not an after-thought adaptively, but actually an interactive prelude of adaptations focused on communicating, assessing, and negotiating levels of parental investment, a jockeying for position leading up to the most important reproductive decision that both partners will make—whether or not they will invest in a child after it is born. This scenario seems to be supported by the interactive quality of female and male hormonal responses during pregnancy—specifically the operation of the HPA axis (the hypothalamic-pituitary-adrenal axis)—as well as behavior during the pregnancy and post-partum. Storey found that men with greater numbers of couvade symptoms had higher hormone levels that correlated with their partners, indicating the possibility of synchronization between male and female responses. This translated into affect and behavior for men with couvade symptoms as these men reported higher levels of anxiety, but also greater feelings of contentment with the pregnancy.* Other studies have shown that couvade symptoms in men are also associated with a higher degree of preparation for fatherhood,† as well as a greater degree of infant caretaking in the postpartum period.‡ For women, as Alison Fleming showed, high levels of cortisol was the best predictor of the quality of maternal care postpartum. High levels of cortisol, as suggested by C. Sue Carter, also seem to be a precursor or potentiator of bonding

* A. E. Storey, C. J. Walsh, R. L. Quinton, and K. E. Wynne-Edwards, "Hormonal Correlates of Paternal Responsiveness in New and Expectant Fathers," *Evolution and Human Behavior* (in press).

† D. C. Longobucco and M. S. Freston, "Relation of Somatic Symptoms to Degree of Paternal Role Preparation of First Time Expectant Fathers," *Journal of Obstetrics, Gynecology, Neonatal Nursing* 18, no. 6 (1989): pp. 487–488.

‡ R. L. Munroe and R. H. Munroe, "Male Pregnancy Symptoms and Cross-Sex Identity in Three Societies," *Journal of Social Psychology* 84 (1971): pp. 11–25.

mechanisms in mammals. What are the implications? Perhaps the signaling feedback between partners and resulting synchronization of the male and female HPA axes helps maintain a positive endocrine environment, the stability of the pair bond, and higher levels of parental investment?

Is there a bigger picture than this? Is there a global view that integrates the endocrinology and behavior of all of pregnancy's participants? I am ending on a highly speculative note, but perhaps what I've been discussing as a dialog of adaptations between pregnant mother and expectant father really should be thought of as a "tri-alogue" of common and conflicting interests of the mother, father, and fetus. After all where does all of this elevated HPA activity start? From the fetus. The mother's endocrine response to her pregnancy is kicked off and partly maintained by lactogenic hormones from the placenta. Thus, through the placenta the fetus has the opportunity to mediate the mother's maternal response, including the state of her "mind."

The fetus's initiation of endocrine activity in the mother early in the pregnancy, which includes an elevated stress response, may also trigger what I will call a "biological program" in the mother to "test" the environment for the level of support her pregnancy will receive. Anxiety, vigilance, elevated emotions, and increased sociability are "probes" that represent the common interest of the fetus and the mother to get as much support as possible. As I said earlier, female symptoms may be a form of signaling. Symptoms at one point in the pregnancy may signal the physiological state of the pregnancy; perhaps at another point, the psychological state of the mother. Both are important pieces of information, and both may be part of determining the father's interest, as well as the level of interest from female kin and the communal group.

Positive responses to the mother's probing of the environment for support, including sympathetic signaling from the father, results in positive changes on the part of both parents during pregnancy and postpartum. Negative feedback, on the other hand, could trigger another set of mechanisms, showing how interests diverge and how counter adaptations may have arisen between mother and fetus. The fetus's interest is to promote its viability no matter what. However, the mother has to evaluate her position and her options throughout the pregnancy. One option may be spontaneous abortion or miscarriage. We tend to think of miscarriage as associated with some genetic malformation, however, at least one study indicates there are correlations between miscarriages and the degree of support and risk in the environment.* Other options are depression and threatened defection—bargaining tools to increase the level of investment from the father and others in the social group.

Essentially, the physiological state of any one member of the "family" during pregnancy might be correlated with the other two. Certainly this would seem to be the case with the mother, that is, the mother's affect is directly influenced by the fetus and the father. The relationship between the fetus and the father is obviously indirect, however, I think a case could be made for mutual influence. The father's behavior could be influenced by the fetus's input into the mother's behavior. Conversely, the fetus, collecting endocrinological "data" through the placenta (of which maternal affect and environment would be a component), could certainly be affected by the father's relationship with the mother. Perhaps the timing of parturition could be an example. Many biologists believe the maturation

---

*J. Olsen, O. Basso, and K. Christensen, "Male Factors and Socioeconomic Indicators Correlate with the Risk of Spontaneous Abortion," *Journal of Obstetrics and Gynaecology*, Bristol (1999).

nd the resultant release of fetal cortisol may
* As Richard Brown has suggested, "there is
iming of human pregnancy. . . . One vari-
or presence of the father."†
ms arose in the social and ecological envi-
s, teasing out the underlying reasons for
with couvade may be difficult. But as a
see them operate in our own behaviors
or and assess their mates during preg-
Do men signal their intentions? I can't
Joseph, my friends who are doctors.
h was unhappy because he felt that
f the emotional process. Meanwhile,
an evolutionary perspective—was carefully watching Joseph, looking for signs that he was identifying with her pregnancy. To her mind his missing her OB appointments and being sullen, critical, and emotionally withdrawn were not exactly the signals of paternal investment and care she was looking for.

What does all this tell us about reproduction, parenting, and human nature in general?

What we think of sentimentally as the family is also an interrelated and dynamic biological system, orchestrating relationships between individuals who have both dependent and independent interests. Supporting and shaping this system are communicative mechanisms between all members that are physiological, emotional, and adaptive.

Against the backdrop of evolutionary give-and-take, I think the

*Gareth Leng, personal communication.
†Richard Brown, *New Scientist*, December 12, 1998.

implications of a paternal response are clear, even if the mechanisms are not. Fortunately, it also means that men's importance to reproduction can be proven to extend beyond being sperm delivery systems. Ultimately, and in the not too distant future, understanding the importance of men to the family at a cellular level will restore men fully to the story of human reproduction. Men are an integral part of the biological system of the family. Our hormonal response to pregnancy is about behavior, not physical function. This hormonal response and the behavior it supports evolved in response to our own reproductive needs as well as the needs of our partners and our children. The behavior it supports is precisely the point. Men's behavior is critical to women's behavior. As David Gubernick points out, "The evidence is clearest for humans. The nature of the emotional relationship between husband and wife affects paternal and maternal behavior. Affectionate and communicative marital relations are associated with sensitive mothering, and mother's feeding competence, and marital harmony is positively related to approval and physical affection shown by both parents towards their children." The fact that we don't give birth does not mean we aren't important to the birth process; the timing and ease of the delivery; the mental state of the mother postpartum; the quality, intensity, and nature of the mother's care; and the eventual success of the child's development.

And even as we are part of the biological circle of the family, we also have a permanent physiological and psychological transformation to call our own. Fatherhood marks us forever, in what we care about, the choices we make, and the intensity and quality of our love.

In a culture where men have been removed from the family scene for hundreds of years, this type of information is revolutionary.

MONTH NINE

THE "RING OF FIRE"

Something is dreadfully wrong.

Julie, who is now so huge that her belly precedes the rest of her body by at least fifteen minutes, is lumbering around hanging curtains, moving furniture, stacking cases of diapers. She is a cartoon of productivity, covering several miles each day without leaving the house. The only reason a painter is doing the baby's room is that the cantilever of Julie's belly makes ladder climbing impossible. Occasionally, when her course takes her past our bedroom, she'll stop to stare balefully at her husband who is languishing supine on the bed, giving a passable imitation of the nearly expired.

I can't move. No, I don't mean tired and sluggish—I did that last week. I mean a narcoleptic fog is rising up from my bone marrow. I mean my blood cells are riding around in miniature Barcaloungers. The other day I was running with the boys around Prospect Park when I just dropped off the back of the pack and stopped, gasping. I felt like I was breathing fluid and not air. My brain stared down at my unresponsive legs, wondering whether they belonged on some other organism, say a turtle. The world looked the same, but I felt oddly different, as if I was wearing a form-fitting aquarium.

The amount of activity going on in the house only made the situation worse. Lauren, our friend, Peace Corps volunteer, and hero of the blood-and-guts birth performance in a regional health clinic in Africa, had been visiting. After a day of social pleasantries, she announces that we have our apartment configured all wrong in her opinion. We should really swap out several rooms, turning Julie's office into a play area for Olivia, and consolidating her work area with mine. The immediate difficulty would be amply compensated for by convenience once the baby arrived. Yeah, well after two straight days of moving tables, sofas, bookcases, credenzas, and home office equipment while fighting what feels like a fatal case of fatigue, I am ready to call it quits forever and hurl myself onto a funeral pyre of our furniture. On the third day I am happy to see our house guest go—back to Africa and her remote hill village where she will no longer pose a danger to Western civilization.

We are talking terminal torpor, lethal lethargy, lassitude bordering on lifelessness. It takes me forever to get up in the morning, and after a few hours of desultory consciousness and a few pathetic attempts to conduct business, all I feel like doing is going back to bed. I can see how and why ancestral men might have taken to their beds before their wives gave birth. That is if I or my wife could accept couvade symptoms as an explanation for what is going on. Judging from her gaze, which all but says "malingerer," a case of sympathetic signaling isn't going to cut it. At this point, it had better be a major terminal disease or multiorgan system failure. How about a quick case of chronic fatigue syndrome?

The consensus is Lyme disease.

"You know, I can't believe this," she says one day. "I'm going to give birth in three weeks and you're the one that can't get out of bed. I can't take any more of this. I want you to see a doctor. You must have Lyme disease. If you don't, I'm going to kill you."

The next day Julie's on her way to one of her regular OB appointments, and I'm on my way to see my GP. What Julie says makes sense. In the last three weeks we have visited Julie's parents' country house in rural Connecticut, my parents in upstate New York, and her aunt and uncle in the Hamptons, all tick-infested areas.

Except my GP is not having any part of it. "It's nothing. You're stressed."

"What are you trying to tell me? That it's all in my head?"

I might be able to accept this from a normal human being, but the first thing you should know is that my GP is always telling me that I'm having psychosomatic symptoms. This I can't figure out. It's not like I'm a hypochondriac. I see the guy once, maybe twice a year, usually with goo coming out of my upper orifices. Would he say the same thing if I showed up with sucking chest wounds? The second thing you should know is that my nickname for the guy is Hamlet, Prince of Denmark. If anyone's manically depressed and imagining things here it's him, not me.

"Let's just say it's your present life circumstances," he says.

"Well, that may be, but I'm telling you right now, I'm not leaving your office until you draw blood."

That seems to do the trick. With a resigned sigh he reaches for his syringe, and one needle stick later I'm out the door and headed across town to Dr. Spyros's to meet Julie. When I get there, Julie's already in the exam room. After a particularly engrossing cervical exam we retire to Spyros's office for a conference to discuss the due date, etcetera. In the middle of a hot and heavy discussion about cervical effacement, Julie ambushes me.

"I'm really worried about Gordon."

"Oh God," I'm thinking, "here we go."

"Go ahead, tell Dr. Spyros what's been going on," she says to me.

So I tell her the whole story—the unshakable lethargy, the turtle legs, the aquarium suit—of my horizontal existence and end it with my one great hope: "I'm really sure it's Lyme disease."

From behind her desk, Spyros starts laughing. I'm utterly humiliated. I'm so humiliated my testicles are retracting. No, they're shrinking and retracting at the same time. At the point when I've got the gonads of a ten-year-old, she finally stops.

"Sometimes men have these reactions," she says, once she's partially regained her composure. "Let's try something," she says, still searching for self-control, but trying her best to be supportive.

A few minutes later I'm heading out the door with prescription for Valium and a firm conviction that God is an angry woman.

I fill the prescription, but I feel funny about taking them. They are somehow symbolic of my abject state and the possibility of some yet-to-be-determined inner failure. I leave the bottle untouched on my bedside table.

Two days later the Lyme test comes back negative. But it doesn't matter. The symptoms are already gone.

Now that I'm back to my perky self, there's a lot to do. My nesting instinct seems to be a little different from that of most men. Whereas the cliché is that most expectant fathers do something to the baby's room, my mania for preparation takes the form of cooking. All joking aside, it makes a lot of sense, in fact it's the first sensible thought I've had. I figure that after the baby's born we are not going to be in any shape to cook meals. So I intend to fill our freezer with easy-to-prepare-and-reheat provisions.

I cook for days. Luckily it's late summer, the perfect time for harvesting and storing food. Wearing my apron, gazing out over our kitchen table heaped with fresh produce, and with pots bubbling on the stove, I feel like a Sicilian *nonna,* or grandmother. I make up pasta sauces in great batches. An acre of barely cooked plum tomatoes is milled into a sauce that can be easily doctored for each meal. Dozens of zucchini hardly larger than fingerlings are laboriously sliced and sautéed with cardamom and ginger into a semiliquid state. My food processor burns out after being fed bush after bush of basil to make pesto. For variety, I concoct several varieties of pea and bean stews that can be served over beds of rice. As a treat, a large stockpot full of French lamb stew bubbles away on a back burner—made mostly with neck bones to gain that velvety marrow. When I'm done, the sight of the white, pearlescent containers stacked neatly in the freezer, ready to hop down and jump into the pot, is pure satisfaction. I estimate we have enough for three months.

Then for the nights when even turning a knob or pushing a button will be too much to bear, I make up a list of the best Chinese, Indian, and pizza takeout restaurants in the neighborhood and stick it on the fridge door.

You have to love a due date. There's nothing like it to make a person get down to business. To have the amorphous feelings of change that have been engulfing me for the last eight months replaced with a sense of imminent finality is a relief. I say imminent finality, but what I really mean is the imminent future. The knowledge that my life is going to be inexorably different within a month is beginning to feel good.

Knowing that our life is changing gives us the chance to view each other in a different light, to present glimpses of our transforming selves to the other in an almost ritual fashion. I am so proud of the way Julie is taking command of life. I have never seen her so sure of herself, so certain of what must be done. Her arches are falling and she waddles when she walks, but her bearing is that of a great general on the eve of battle. Miltiades at Marathon. Henry V at Agincourt. Wellington at Waterloo.

Meanwhile I am in the kitchen. But I'm proud of that, too. It seems like a little thing, an obvious thing, and maybe even a slightly pathetic thing, but being able to think about our new life, to anticipate not just my needs but Julie's needs and the needs of someone who isn't even quite here yet, has been, as they say, a huge paradigm shift. My love of cooking also puts me in touch with the sense of nurturing I'm going to need to use. After all, in my own way, I've been feeding Olivia *in utero* for nearly nine months. Sometimes I feel like I'm building a huge cocoon of food around Julie and Olivia. I call it "fruiting the nut."

This explicit teamwork, with each of us contributing something particular to a goal, feels good—as well as makes me occasionally wonder what we've been doing until now in our married lives. But never mind, I'm building on the feeling, taking on other projects where I can contribute something particular and valuable.

Like hiring a nanny. Searching for and arranging child care has got to be one of the most perverse challenges a soon-to-be parent faces. Consider it one of the hallmarks of our times that most of us can't be assured of the type of care that our babies will receive because we actually can't be present for much of it. Transfer this anxiety to a situation where we know absolutely nothing about taking care of newborns and yet have to choose the ideal person to provide it. The only appropriate thing to do is to focus all this two-career yuppie guilt onto the process.

Neither Julie nor I has ever really hired anybody to do anything, so we mutually decide that I should take on the role of interviewer, since I am the more socially assertive and ruder of the two of us. I call up our Harvard MBA friend Miranda for advice. She just happens to have a list of thirty questions that she routinely asks when interviewing baby-sitter candidates and faxes it over to me. The questions range from "What does your partner do for a living?" (establishes what their home life is like, Miranda explains) to "Do you have any religious affiliations?" (you want to weed out the wackos who want to convert your baby) to "How much television do you watch?" (you want your baby-sitter interacting with your kid, not teaching it to watch TV). Some of these questions are strategically brilliant, but I decide that I'm only rude enough to ask about ten, and then toss in a few of my own. We place an add in the *Irish Echo*, which is for historical reasons the baby-sitter-advertising newspaper in New York, and within days the calls start coming in. Most of the women who answer the ad are from the Caribbean Islands and live across the park in Flatbush.

Choosing is difficult. Everyone is smart and personable. All are staunch, upstanding churchgoers. Initially we are drawn to a woman named Diane because of her verve, but our sentimental favorite is Margaret. She had for years worked in the laundry at the bottom of our street, where we had struck up a casual acquaintance with her as we dropped off and picked up our clothing. One day we passed by to see the laundry shuttered and workman removing the machines. Other than the inconvenience of having to find a new laundry, we thought nothing of it, until Cecilia, our neighbor and Julie's best friend, mentioned that she had run into Margaret and that Margaret was in desperate straits as her job had disappeared without warning. Cecilia, ever kind and resourceful, had taken her number on a whim and now passed it along to us. So we decided to interview Margaret. She had few child care references, but she had raised three children of her own, and she showed remarkable initiative, offering to take a baby CPR course before she came to work for us.

In the end we decided to go with Margaret. Our reasons were almost ineffable. What we really liked about her is that we feel so relaxed in her presence. Being with Margaret is like stepping into the cool serenity of a church on a hot day. The way we figure it, she has two qualities we lack and will need most over the next few months, if not years—faith and calm.

"The 1000XL is truly the Gold Standard in breast pumps today."

Jose, a rep from a maternal care supply company, has traveled all the way from the Upper West Side of Manhattan to deliver and explain the virtues of his product. There seems something slightly incongruous about a twenty-something male knowing more about the workings of Julie's breasts than either Julie or me, but at this point in our journey I am so accustomed to incongruity that I am unruffled.

The machine itself, however, is something out of a nightmare. It looks like a miniature oil refinery or an electric utility power plant, replete with pistons and piping. A transparent plastic tube snakes upward to a Y-fitting, splitting off to two soft plastic cones that fit over the breasts. Jose flips a switch and with a slow wheeze the machine starts its pneumatic suckling. It is what it looks and sounds like: a milking machine designed by the best minds of the nineteenth century. I want to cover it with a tea cozy. Given the demand for this sort of thing these days you'd think the manufacturers would get with it and learn a thing or two from fashion and science. Commission Jean-Paul Gaultier to design the housing and the accessories, and then put a chip in it to record and play back your own baby's cries. You know, infant cues, milk letdown, etcetera.

After Jose leaves, Julie takes off her shirt and bra and performs an impromptu lactation dance, shuffling around the room holding the suction cups to her breasts, transparent tubes trailing.

It's going to be a brave new world, and it seems like much of it is going to be attached to Julie's breasts. I'm not sure we're ready for it. What have we come to that we have to be reintroduced to our own bodies? There are some evenings, when I'm not comparing Julie's belly to Macchu Picchu, that I lay next to her and marvel at her breasts. Often as not, I catch Julie also staring at them. Sometimes our hands meet as we measure their heft. How full they have become. How dark the aureoles. I count the Montgomery tubercules. When I squeeze the nipples a tiny bead of clear liquid emerges into the light.

For men, women's breasts are the pleasure toggles in the sexual cockpit. Any other function is Oedipal foul territory. Even women seem somewhat wary about their functional purpose. There seems to be as much worry among women of my acquaintance about mammary plasticity—as in "Will they return to their former perky selves?"—as there is concern about their efficacy as nutritional fonts.

The other day we attended our first lactation class, held in a dilapidated community center in Greenwich Village. About twenty couples attended. It was late in the afternoon, so everyone was still in corporate work suits. The women carried baby dolls to use as props for practicing positioning techniques. What struck me most was not the sense of vestigial irrelevance and discomfort felt by the men—this has become all too common a feeling to even bother recording. Instead what I noted (with some carefully concealed amusement) was that the women seemed to have exactly the same feelings.

This was not lost on our instructor, a woman who, while in the

Gaia endomorph mold, was not warm and embracing. She actually seemed a little exasperated and a tad resentful. I suspect it was because she, too, had picked up the carrier wave of lactional alienation and unease generated by the women in the room. After a little pep talk—the tone of which I think I can describe as St. Mammaria among the sinners—she started us off on some truly awful instructional videotapes.

My eyes repelled by the homemade production values, I scanned the room, having little else to do but breathe. The reptilian male part of my brain generated some idle thoughts. Why are the forces of good always a little dull, underpaid, badly dressed, inherit shabby interior decoration, and a little resentful because of it? Okay, all kidding aside. Why does everything about reproduction always have to be so symbolic? Why can't it be just a process? Why does everything have to be a belief system? I mean here we are at the cusp of the twenty-first century and our instructor has turned herself into a High Priestess of Lactation to get her point across. On the other hand, I can kind of see her point. Her audience is a room full of reluctant career women who are uncomfortable with their bodies, uncomfortable with their new roles, uncomfortable with nature and their natures.

As my eyes drift across the room, something jars my semidozing brain. One of the women has brought as her breast-feeding prop not a baby doll, but a stuffed rabbit. Now that's a statement. Either this woman has been driven completely insane, or she has achieved the perfect attitude.

We're now officially late. Due day comes and goes without incident, not even a lousy Braxton-Hicks contraction. I was hoping for a big Hollywood moment with Julie faltering in mid-stride or mid-sentence and saying, "Gordon, this is it," preferably at a convenient time, say after breakfast. I could catch her in mid-swoon and whisk her off to the hospital, leaving the dishes unwashed on the table. But, nothing.

Oddly enough, being late isn't really an anxious feeling. It's not like the Roadrunner cartoon where the Coyote overshoots the curve and hangs in space before plummeting. It's not like being a space shuttle pilot and having a launch postponed because of the weather. It's more like the feeling that the Tibetan teacher Norbu Rinpoche, who was always famously late to his lectures, once described. The feeling you want in meditation, he would say, is the feeling you have between the time he's supposed to be there and the time he actually arrives.

Being late feels like a little free time before enlightenment. It feels like we've unplugged from one life and are waiting to be plugged into another. Everything else has been suspended. The clients have been notified. The social engagements have been canceled. The paint is drying. The fax machine and the phones are still.

Actually that's not true. The phone rings constantly. Our friends are driving us crazy. All day long they've been calling. "Did anything happen yet?" I'm not sure what stupid answer I should give. "Yes, Julie's having contractions two minutes apart but we've been waiting to hear from you before we go to the hospital," to "Yes, we've had the child already, but we're hiding it in the closet." I had no idea that being loved could be this irritating.

Plus we're running up against a variable we hadn't really expected. August is not the month to have babies. Everyone, including our doctors, is away on vacation or at least spending their weekends at the beach. Spyros tried to break it to us as early as possible that she and her partner Balakian would be trading weekends throughout August until Labor Day. When both of them starting sharing weekend coverage with another set of OBs across town, Drs. Lee and Benegar, it became even more complicated. So we dutifully schlep into Manhattan and the Upper West Side to meet them and drop off our birth plans. They are nice enough. Lee takes a few moments between appointments to chat. Benegar smiles brightly and shakes our hands, barely breaking stride as she passes briskly from one exam room to another. It doesn't feel reassuring; it feels like the lottery.

Spyros also tells us we have ten days to produce Olivia or she's going to induce. We put in calls to our support crew. Erica suggests lots of sex to jump-start things. Susan votes for nipple-sucking and stimulation to get the oxytocin going. Someone else opts for really spicy food. We try all three—sometimes independently, sometimes in combination. Mostly, we try to spend quiet time together. We turn on the air conditioner and just lie like lumps on the bed, enjoying our last few days in the walled garden.

JULIE: I'm having some contractions.

GORDON: I'm really tired. Please don't have the baby in the next eight hours.

JULIE: Let's time them.

GORDON: You must be kidding. They're not strong enough to time.

JULIE: How would *you* know how strong they are? *You* are not the one having them.

GORDON: I know, because if they were really strong you wouldn't be wolfing down half your body weight in watermelon right now.

• • •

Julie woke me up at 3 A.M. to announce the arrival of the "mucous plug," which she thoughtfully preserved in a hank of tissue. Of all the signs and auguries of the last month, this one is actually significant. Finally, something is happening. Julie's cervix has snorted out the gob of snot that has kept the uterus sealed off from the world. We both stare down at it. It looks huge, about the size of a quarter, and gooily profound in the weak light, like a dark nebula of aged blood and albumen. A day or two later we drag it out again in daylight to stare at its wondrous, mummified remains.

The worst possible thing has happened.

Julie woke me at 1 A.M. to tell me she'd been having contractions for the last hour during which I'd been in a deep beery sleep. I've been working late into the evening for several days to revise some projects that had to be changed after I thought they were approved, so I'm exhausted. Tonight, we went out for Korean—the spicy food thing—and I had a few beers to relax. Nothing had happened for a few days and I thought it was safe. A few beers, some great food, a good night's sleep, and I'm ready for anything. What a mistake. Damn beers. Damn food.

I had long fantasized that I would do and say the perfect things when this moment arrived. Instead all I can offer is a mumbled "Try to go back to sleep," as my brain utters a prayer that this is just a false alarm, otherwise, we're fucked. I turn my sleeping body toward Julie, to keep an eye on her just in case.

Except she can't go back to sleep. Every once in a while I pop an eye open and I see Julie doing some controlled breathing. She's too jacked up on adrenaline and the contractions are too painful. Several checks later, she's gone. I sleep-walk to the bathroom to find her sitting backward on the toilet. I tell her to come back into the bedroom, but she wants to stay in the bathroom. It's more comfortable. She looks very lonely.

I go back to the bedroom feeling awful and useless, but I've got to get a little sleep or I'm going to be more than useless. This certainly wasn't the way I imagined it was going to happen.

At 6:30 A.M. I put in a call to Susan, our labor doula. She arrives around 9 A.M. and takes over. What a relief. Feeling absolutely shattered, I go upstairs into the parlor and crash on the couch. After a couple of hours of fitful sleep I feel better. I come downstairs to find Julie laboring in the kitchen. She's sitting backward on a kitchen chair vocalizing into the air. Susan's standing behind her massaging her neck. Julie looks up and seems happy to see me. Thank God. I take turns with Susan massaging Julie's back and neck. Putting counter pressure on Julie's lower back during the contractions seems to help a little with the pain. When it's not my turn, I wash dishes or putter with food. I cut up a perfectly ripe cantaloupe and feed it to Julie, shoving the juicy chunks into her mouth with my fingers.

The next hours pass in what seems an idyll. The kitchen seems to be the perfect birth chamber. Sun streams in from the bank of windows overlooking the garden. Outside, butterflies circle the last of the yellow rose's crumbling blooms. In the tiny bathroom directly off the kitchen, Julie soaks in the tub and gossips and trades stories with Susan, who is sitting on the toilet seat. How they met their husbands, etcetera. A little later I make lunch, some leftover chicken soup and a small, perfectly dressed salad. Susan compliments the food, and I open the freezer to show off my stash. We all have a laugh. When the contractions come, Julie changes position on the chair and Susan presses on her back.

With Julie roaring in the air, it sounds a little like a game park. Then I switch to a more pastoral channel. I suddenly have a vision of pregnant women laboring in Prospect Park, walking beneath the great elms with their partners, pausing to groan on the park benches, their vocalizing converging into harmonies while runners and bikers and the rest of normal life whiz by.

Back to real life. In a flash, six hours have passed since Susan arrived. It's now 3 P.M. Julie has been laboring for fourteen hours. The contractions are irregular, ranging from ten to fifteen minutes apart, but they are very painful. Julie says she feels "very open." We all consult for a moment and decide to put in a call to the hospital. By now we know it isn't going to be Spyros. We check our notes. Dr. Benegar. We put in our call, and Susan and then Julie talk to her. Benegar seems anxious and not at all reassuring. The first call is inconclusive, but ten minutes later the phone rings and it's Benegar again. She wants us to come in so she can check Julie's cervix.

I can tell that Susan thinks it's too early. I, too, feel unease and foreboding. But what can we do? We don't want to pass along our fears to Julie. She's already in a lot of pain, and I can tell that she's picking up on our misgivings and that it's making her more tense. Hey, maybe we'll get lucky. Maybe we'll get to the hospital and Julie will be at seven centimeters.

At 3:30 P.M. we finally leave for the hospital. Susan takes Julie out, while I scoop up our stuff. The last thing I grab as I head out the door is the purple Eddie Bauer gym bag. The unfiltered light outside is dazzling and surreal. I can't say it feels good to leave our home. I bring the car around, a little red Honda, and we pack Julie into it. It's a forty-minute drive from Park Slope to Lenox Hill Hospital. On Flatbush Avenue, a family crosses the street in front of us against the light. It looks like a closer call than it is. I have plenty of time to stop, but the braking tugs us all a little forward. Susan says, "Let's try to get to the hospital without killing any innocent bystanders," to which I reply, "We would only be completing the cosmic circle of life and death." Apparently she doesn't think it's funny.

We continue on over the Brooklyn Bridge and the FDR Drive without incident. The Honda is silent. Julie has her head buried in Susan's lap. Susan is busy burrowing her hands into the small of Julie's back. I'm driving with the detached calm that comes when you feel like you're playing your part in the destined order of things—my thoughts everywhere and nowhere.

Lenox Hill has got to be one of the richest and best hospitals in the world, but it is still a hospital. Hospitals are temples to our role in entropy. Step into the lobby and you smell putrefaction stemmed with Lysol and betadine. The guard at the elevator kindly offers us a wheelchair. Susan immediately says no, and I can tell that although we look like characters stumbling along in a Beckett play, she wants to maintain our own pace and control.

The nurses in Labor and Delivery are efficient. Within ten minutes or so we're in an exam room and Julie's being checked by a resident, a blond woman with the personality of a chest freezer. "Great," I'm thinking, "the first member of the medical corps we meet is a member of the walking dead." Soon she renders a verdict: two centimeters, maybe three centimeters, at position +1. "Plus one" means that the baby's head is one centimeter past the midline of the pelvis and "engaged" in the pelvic opening. Susan and I look at each other. We both look at Julie. Julie looks crushed. A few minutes later Dr. Benegar walks in and confirms the resident's exam. Even worse, she places the position at −1, meaning that the baby's head is still not engaged. She puts an external monitor on Julie. For the first time we hear Olivia, a steady tom-tom-tom at a perfect 140 beats per minute. For a few moments we listen transfixed and mesmerized. And renewed.

Benegar turns to me. She wants to give Julie a "hep-lock" (a plastic port that keeps a vein open so that medication can be administered quickly) and start an IV with fluids. I choose my words carefully, but she seems a little taken aback when I tell her I'm not in favor of it at this time.

"You've read our birth plan? We would like every opportunity to have an unassisted birth if possible."

"It's only a precautionary measure. If something goes wrong, or if we decide to go ahead with painkillers and induce the baby, the vein is already open."

"I understand your concerns, but I think we're very early on in this process. At this point I don't think there's any reason to believe that we can't progress on our own, and I don't think a hep-lock and an IV will have the desired psychological effect on my wife."

"I really think you should think about it. We don't want to fumble around trying to get an IV into your wife in case there's an emergency."

"So far everything seems normal. A hep-lock can be painful. I don't want it distracting from what's going on. Can we revisit this in a couple of hours?"

Benegar agrees, reluctantly. I can tell that she isn't too happy about the situation, but I've tried to be as diplomatic as possible while standing my ground. It's now 5 o'clock in the afternoon. The only good news we've had so far is that business is light and we can go right to the delivery room, instead of having to wait our turn in one of the labor rooms. While the room is being readied, the nurses suggest that we "ambulate."

So we become refugees wandering the halls of the sixth floor. Julie shuffling along with Susan and me on either side of her. We immediately understand why so many people advised against going to the hospital for as long as possible. We feeel neither here nor there, occupying some nether world of perpetual fluorescent green twilight. Groups of people on their way to somewhere walk by and momentarily stare at us. Occasionally we pass by the nursery on our rounds. The neat rows of babies wailing silently behind the inch-thick plate glass seem a world away.

Compared to the labor rooms, the delivery room is the Hilton among Super–8s. It's big and it has its own bathroom and shower. We set ourselves up and try to make ourselves at home. It doesn't feel like home but it's infinitely better than the hallways.

Julie's hungry. It's against medical protocol, but Susan reaches into her bag and pulls out half a tuna fish sandwich and sneaks it to Julie. Later I go out for a fried egg sandwich and bring it back. The warm yolky smell instantly permeates the room and humanizes it. It's impossible to miss, but the nurses seem unconcerned.

Benegar comes in around 7 o'clock and checks Julie again. Nothing has happened. Julie's still between two and three centimeters dilated. Again Benegar asks to install a hep-lock. We have a brief conference and again I decline. I can tell that she's just shy of being exasperated with me, but since there is no medically necessary reason for doing the procedure, there is little she can insist on.

After she leaves, I turn to Susan. What do we do? Julie's condition is deteriorating. She's been up laboring now for nineteen hours. She's missed a night's sleep. The contractions, while irregular and unproductive, are still becoming increasingly painful. Susan suggests taking Julie into the shower to try and relax her.

She also suggests some nipple stimulation as a way of accelerating the process.

I have my doubts, but there is little else to do. Just waiting around is much too grim. I reach into my gym bag, put on a swimsuit, and take Julie into the shower. I sit her down on a stool and run the water. She is shivering. Her legs and back are tense. I start off by giving her a massage. Eventually the bathroom warms up and Julie stops shaking. I bend down and suck her nipples for what seems like an eternity. Occasionally I look up. I can barely see her face because of the fog. Julie has her eyes shut and is elsewhere. We seem lost.

At 9:30 P.M. Benegar checks Julie again. It's not good news. She's only at four centimeters. Benegar and Marjorie, our nurse, both stare intently at the external monitor readout and shake their heads. The contractions are not strong enough, regular enough, or frequent enough to be productive. Yet, for Julie, they are getting more painful. Her vocalizing, which until an hour ago had sounded directed and asserted, now has taken on a tremulous ululating quality. It's hard to tell who's in control, Julie or the pain. Also, Julie's membranes have ruptured sometime between Benegar's last exam and this one.

I can tell that Benegar wants to talk to me again and I signal her that I want to talk to Julie and Susan alone for a moment. "Maybe you can hang on for another couple of hours until the next examination," I tell Julie. She doesn't answer right away, and I can tell she's reached her limit. She looks awful, ashen, and wrung out. Julie turns to Susan and says, "I feel confused." Susan reassures her that whatever she wants will be the right decision. Julie says, "I think I need some help."

There is a strange moment when you give yourself over to the

system. Up until this point I had viewed Benegar with a slight attitude of suspicion. None of this, however, was her fault. Our first
problem was we didn't know her. Our second problem was that she
was the product of a culture whose interests, methods, and ideas
did not always correspond with the ones we had adopted. Ideally,
we had hoped that we wouldn't really need her. The birth might be
difficult, but it would progress, and she would participate mini
mally at the end.

Now that Julie's body had stalled we needed to bring Benegar
into the loop. Instead of a potential adversary, I now had to trust
her and approach her as an ally. "What are our next steps?" I
asked. "What can we do incrementally that can help Julie along
and still keep our goals in the picture?" The answer was Demerol
to kill the pain, followed by a pitocin drip to try and regularize
the contractions and fully efface the cervix. If that happens,
maybe Julie can then push the baby out.

I relayed the information to Julie and Susan. Julie agreed, and
our nurse Marjorie got right to work on the IV. She is a gum-
smacking sort who seems straight out of Walker Evans's
Appalachia. As she works, she mutters, "Yep, during my first birth I
had the Demerol first to take the edge off and then moved on to
the epidural." She says all this as calmly as a person reaching for a
six-pack of Bud. Later when I ask her where she's from she tells me,
"Bay Ridge, Brooklyn." Now she turns to Benegar: "Should we 'pit'
her?" Benegar nods and then injects the Demerol into the IV.
Almost immediately Julie says, "It tastes so sweet," and then she is
asleep. Susan curls up in a chair, and I roll out my foam mat and lie
down on the floor.

The last thing I remember is looking up and seeing Julie on
all fours. Even while her brain is asleep, her body is reacting to

the force of the contractions. One hand raises upward as if she is climbing an invisible ladder.

The plan isn't working. It's midnight, Saturday. Twenty-four hours since Julie's contractions began. The Demerol has worn off and she's awake. She's still only four to five centimeters open and the pain from the pitocin-driven contractions is horrible. She's falling apart, and it's obvious she isn't going to be able to tolerate this. She asks for an epidural.

Thirty very long minutes later a tall thin guy in a lab coat with a very unassuming air produces himself at our doorway and announces: "Hi! I'm Rob the Epidural Man!" I am prepared for just about everything except friendliness, but his manner is a relief. He shakes my hand hard, and tells me he is going to need my help. He has Julie bend herself into a ball, spreading her vertebrae apart. "I'm going to need you to hold your wife's head firmly onto her chest. Both of you stay absolutely still. This is really important. Make sure she does not move."

He says this all in a friendly, almost offhand manner, but then again someone who is about to snake a needle into your partner's vertebral canal doesn't need to do much to command attention. Epidurals are tricky. Rob the anesthesiologist has to guide the needle through a muscle wall and then past the outer sheet of the dural lining—a strong, thick membrane composed of dense fibrous tissue—into the epidural space. He has to do this without going too far and penetrating the inner dural lining, which is millimeters away from the spinal nerves. And he has to do it all by feel.

As Rob works, I can hear Marjorie of Bay Ridge by way of the Smokies chewing gum and talking to Benegar. She's telling Benegar that she's afraid I'm going to pass out. Doesn't she have anything better to do than think? Ten minutes later Rob is done and away with a big wave. I'm sorry to see him go. Benegar tells me that she is going to give Julie some oxygen to keep blood gas levels up and that she wants to switch from external to internal monitoring. She holds up a thin leader of wire with a small corkscrew hook on the end. I give the go-ahead and Benegar reaches into Julie's vagina and attaches the lead to Olivia's head. There is a moment when the telemetry goes silent. Then the fetal heartbeat returns as normal.

Julie is already asleep and everyone else is clearing out. Susan looks really uncomfortable sleeping in her chair so I give her my foam mat and a blanket. Julie will need her to be fresh and alert and available. As for me, I go out into the night and take a short walk. It feels liberating to be out of the hospital. Even at 2 A.M., New York is going full bore. I stop at a newsstand and buy the Sunday *New York Times* and bring it back to the room.

The doctors and nurses are gone. The labor consultant is tucked in. I watch over my sleeping wife, tend the fire, and brood. I feel fully engaged and ready to keep trying, but I am not optimistic. None of us has given up, but I have to say that I no longer believe things are going to turn out the way Julie wants them to. Things have not gone our way. Julie's labor has stalled and it's quite likely that she is in "back labor." Babies in this position are head down but facing forward, increasing the likelihood that they can get hung up on the lower spine and pelvis. I also know that if Julie can't push this baby out early tomorrow morning, Benegar is going to want a C-section. While Benegar didn't say anything at the time, I knew that as soon as she announced that Julie's membranes had broken at the 9:30 exam, we were on a twelve-hour clock.

I take a moment to commune with my unborn daughter. In the darkness, in my profound fatigue, her presence is palpable to my imagination. The steady tom-tom of her heart is the surest thing I know. Her birth, no matter how it happens, will be a victory.

Then I spread out the sections of the *New York Times* on the floor and go to sleep on them.

When I awake at 7 A.M., my shoulder is so numb from the cold floor, I can't move it right away. There is already a lot of activity in the room. Julie is awake. She actually looks refreshed and fully present. Benegar's also there. She looks like shit, a complete wreck. She's been up all night, no doubt tending other births. Benegar checks Julie's cervix and announces that she's fully dilated. This feels like good news. Marjorie says, in her best white trash accent, "Maybe we should get this show on the road."

It feels like we've made progress, but there are more complications ahead. The contractions have changed from being painful and vague to now being more concentrated and expulsive. The problem is that with the epidural Julie can't really feel them. She tries to push but it all feels unfocused and she can't get into synch. Julie is trying to push by bearing down while she exhales, a technique that is not working for her. After about an hour of this fumbling around Julie looks confused. Susan leans over and they conference for a few minutes. I can hear Susan saying something like: "It doesn't work for everybody. If something's not working it's okay to let it go." Julie says, "Please, tell me what to do."

Julie starts pushing now by holding her breath and bearing down. Susan and I are on both sides of her. We try out different things. Sometimes we pick up Julie's deadened legs. She grasps her thighs, pulls back, and pushes. I watch her face turn from white to purple. Then for a while, we try hauling Julie up into a squatting position with every contraction.

• • •

It's almost ten o'clock. We've been working with Julie now for two hours and nothing is happening. There's a creeping realization that the hard part of the birth, which we thought was behind us, is actually in front of us.

Marjorie's shift is over and a new nurse, Leah, has replaced her. Leah is the complete opposite of Marjorie. She is sweet and soft with a slight Southern accent. She looks like she just stepped out of *Southern Living* magazine. Benegar, who has been in and out all morning checking her other patients, is now with us full-time. I can tell that she's getting anxious about our progress. She sits in her chair and stares disapprovingly at the monitor. During the contractions, Olivia's heartbeat sometimes dips down below 100 beats per minute. As soon as they let up, it jumps back to 140 beats. This is completely normal, but Benegar is watchful for any signs of fetal distress.

Susan suggests that we take Julie out of the bed and have her try a labor stool. This particular suggestion is a disaster. Without feeling below her waist, Julie has no balance, and Susan and I struggle to keep her upright. After a few attempts, we abandon. Then Leah has a suggestion. Let's try it on all fours. Susan is immediately enthusiastic, and we haul Julie over to the bed and put her on her hands and knees. After a few minutes of pushing Julie yells out, "I felt something move!" and the baby seemed to descend for a moment. Then it moves back up, and Julie is despondent. "Why won't she come out?" she cries.

Benegar has reached the end of her patience. From her chair, she keeps talking over the activity, telling Julie that she's got to get the baby out soon. "I'm going to have to do something if things don't start happening." Benegar avoids the C-word, but it's all too obvious what she can do that we can't. Julie loses it and yells at Benegar, "Don't say that to me. It's not helping me. You're making me very anxious. I really don't want to have a C-section! I can do this, but you have to help me."

This seems to break Benegar loose from her chair-bound stupor. Mustering whatever energy she has left, she jumps up and moves to the bedside. "Push hard! That's it, get mad! Get mad at me! Get this baby out!" She has Julie move back to a seated position. She digs her fingers into Julie's perineum to give her a reference point and yells, "There is where I want you to push! Come on now, ready?" We all count to ten in unison, and Julie pushes. The pain is stratospheric. Julie is screaming.

But she's getting the hang of it. Soon we are in a bit of a rhythm. Benegar, Leah, Susan, and I counting, Julie pushing and howling. We keep doing it. It feels right, but after ten minutes or so still nothing has happened. Julie says, "Am I doing something wrong?" Everyone yells back, "No! You're doing it right!" Then Julie says, "Where's the baby?"

Oh, the baby. Benegar looks down and visibly startles. "The baby's head is here!" she yells. Olivia's head, during the span of their short conversation, had actually surfaced at the lips of Julie's vagina.

All hell breaks loose. Things are happening now. People are rushing around Julie's body. Susan is at Julie's head. Leah is near Julie's lower legs. Benegar is in the catcher's position. She's already put on a vinyl apron and is working on moving Julie's perineum past the baby's head. I step away slightly into the background to make room. Leah says to Julie, "Do you want to feel the baby's head?" Julie reaches down past her labial lips, which are engorged and extended like livery rosettes to touch the baby's scalp.

The baby's head crowns. Now comes the ring of fire. Julie is screaming. The four of us are yelling, exhorting her. She screams and pushes. The baby's head moves a centimeter forward with each effort, then recedes half a centimeter. She screams and pushes again. The baby moves forward a little more, then recedes. Benegar is feverishly working on the labia with her gloved hands.

From amid Julie's genitals, which are unfolding like a giant lotus blossom, Olivia's head pops out. I am but a breath away, I see everything. She is awake and alert. Her eyes are wide open. They are two black marbles roving to and fro. Time ratchets forward a notch. Benegar tips Olivia's head to one side and frees a shoulder. Olivia jets out into space followed by a gush of green and black fluid fountaining from the birthspot, covering Benegar. Benegar, moving quickly, cradles her backward with both hands and passes her off to Leah. Another set of hands comes into the frame carrying a blue bulb and suctions mucus from Olivia's nose and throat. Benegar quickly clamps the umbilical cord in two places with hemostats, and then with surgical scissors cuts the cord with an audible *snap!* It is the sound of my mother's Japanese garden shears cutting through iris stems.

All this has occurred in one motion. Only a few seconds have passed. Two extra delivery nurses who have appeared from nowhere place Olivia in an incubator and wave an oxygen wand over her face. I hear a series of tiny staccato hiccups, which turn into coughs, and then a muffled cry that sounds like a muted jazz trumpet. Then she starts crying for real. As her throat clears a tiny crystalline vibrato emerges that's pure Ella Fitzgerald.

"We made a baby!" Julie is yelling. Benegar is still bent over Julie's vagina, holding the umbilicus in one hand and staring at the entrance. She looks like she's ice fishing. She pulls ever so gently and soon a huge purple-red mass appears, oozes out like an octopus from a rock fissure, and slumps into her gloved hands. The placenta has arrived and we look upon it for a moment almost affectionately—Olivia's source of sustenance for these past nine months. Benegar unfurls it and spreads it out to show us where it attached to the uterus wall and to the membrane of the amniotic sac. I imagine it like some great water lily, the leaf like a great palm spread toward the mother-sun. Julie asks to touch it. We both touch it.

Thirty-five hours have passed since Julie's contractions started. The nurses bring us Olivia, now appearing as a freshly scrubbed newborn baby. The placenta is put aside and forgotten. Susan takes Olivia and places her on Julie's chest. Julie keeps repeating, "We made a baby!" For one more moment all of us are converged in the same frame. Benegar, Leah, Susan, Julie, and I all huddled around Olivia, who is beginning to nurse. Then in the next moment everyone disperses. Life is already different. Good-bye, Dr. Benegar. Good-bye, Leah. We will never see you again, but thank you.

Two nurses appear from the newborn nursery with a trolley. It seems too soon, but we give them Olivia. They slowly trundle off. I can't bear being separated so quickly. I look at Julie and Susan. They wave me on. I trail the nurses down the corridors to the nursery. They disappear through the double doors where I can't follow. I move to the plate-glass windows where I can see them place her in a bassinet among the neat rows of bassinets.

I press my face against the walls of the domed city where I continue observing carefully my new life.

EPILOGUE

PREGNANT MEN

Of course the first thing you have to do after giving birth is pack up and leave. After being gently shooed out of the delivery room, we still had forty-eight hours to spend in the hospital, so we decided to splurge and get ourselves a room in the hospital's new private wing, paying for the difference ourselves. Even though the total cost of one of these rooms was about $700 per night, the decor was pure Ethan Allen. Tinny brass doorknobs blinding as a bare light bulb; wall sconces with little mansard hats on them; an entertainment center in the shape of Paul Revere's home. Frankly I preferred the honest sterility of the rest of the hospital.

No matter. We were finally alone, except of course for a small corps of nurses. The way the room was set up, the husband is supposed to sleep in this convertible Barcalounger that folds out into a bed about the width of a tooth. We quickly dispensed with this idea and I joined Julie and Olivia on the full-sized "patient's" bed. The three of us snoozed contentedly through the night until the nurses woke us in the morning. I think they were a little scandalized by the fact that I was in the bed, too. We spent the morning fielding phone calls and receiving friends who were dying to visit. Later I found out that one of the couvade rituals practiced in the Caribbean involves the father, mother, and newborn receiving the rest of the village at bedside. Two days later we went back to Brooklyn.

The truth is that you change and the world remains the same. But that's not how you experience it. To our eyes everything about the world was different. Even our Park Slope apartment was transformed. As we passed through the doorway I could feel the filaments of a chrysalis parting. I'll never forget the feeling of crossing that threshold cradling Olivia in my arms—the lousy apartment of our youth was now a home.

In the cool darkness of our bedroom we lived. Our seclusion was not entirely a matter of happiness. Susan came over to fine-tune Julie's breast-feeding. Julie's nipples had become progressively tender, sore to the point where each feeding session was an endurance. Julie's mood had also skidded into a mild depression. It was subtle and completely normal, but unnerving to both of us. Faithful as a sled dog I took over the chores of the new quotidian. I fetched Olivia at feeding times and brought her to Julie. I bathed her and changed her. I prepared our meals. Occasionally I would go out into the world and shop. Soon Julie's mood lifted and we entered a short halcyon period. Julie's breasts lost their tenderness. Olivia slept peaceably through the night, waking only for her 2 A.M. feeding. Life was perfect for about a month. Then came colic.

The "Gold Standard in breast pumps" didn't work for us. It took Julie forever to fill one of those little plastic sacs. The relentless pneumatic *phfft, phfft* was maddening, especially when the payoff was measured in dribbles. It didn't help that when we confided this to a friend who was also nursing, she threw open her freezer to display her enormous hoard of frozen colostrum. Her bovine pride was unwatchable. So when it came time to start working again and our nanny, Margaret, came on board full-time, we eventually decided to start supplementing with formula. I was delighted. It meant that I could also participate in feeding Olivia. I can still remember that first feeding session, Coach Susan sitting beside me on the couch. She had me stick my finger in Olivia's mouth to understand her suckling reflex. The tug on my finger was profound. I was startled. Its force seemed to come from something much larger than a six-pound being. Once as a child I stepped into a mountain stream after the snowmelt and the rushing water grabbed my leg. I still remember that feeling of almost being swept away.

We're driving down I–84. I can barely see the road, the tears are flowing so generously. I look over at Julie; she's crying a rainforest. We look at each other and laugh and hand each other tissues to fend off the mudslide of mucus that accompanies crying. Year-old Olivia in her car seat closely inspecting a board book is doing her best to ignore yet another instance of our drop-of-the-hat lachrymizing. On the CD player Celine Dion or Tori Amos is singing Brahms's lullaby, part of one of those collections of "celebrities do baby songs." It's awful. It has all the authenticity of an AT&T commercial. But we can't help ourselves. We're parents. A blade of grass grows and we're moved.

I don't know how Julie feels, but as a man I don't always enjoy these oceanic moments. But I'm glad they're there. They are a good reference point for me during these times—an inner badge of passage.

There is not the slightest doubt in my mind that men who

experience pregnancy and birth are marked permanently by a biological transformation. Every man I have ever spoken to about it who has become a father, including many biologists, agrees. We all feel different, and now we know it's because in all likelihood we literally are different. What we think, what we care about, the risks we're willing to take, our capacity for love—all changed.

What value is this information? I'm not sure. Right now we're at a weird juncture in the cultural history of the family. Men have been absent for so long from the circle of day-to-day family operations and intimacies that fatherhood occupies the same niche as folklore. The erosion of the value of "patriarchal" values is so complete that while we have a place at the family table our status is almost that of a guest. And since belief in science as the only legitimizing authority for all reality is our culture's peculiar brand of insanity, the little scientific research that does exist on fathers isn't enough to articulate our importance.

The most important idea to come out of this is that transformation through pregnancy and childbirth is not just purely the woman's domain, with men as a postfeminist add-on. Men become "pregnant," too, in a way that is much more concrete than just metaphor. Men undergo a bodily rite of transformation of their own that is cellular and permanent. The change is not as profound in physiology or purpose, not as large in scale or intensity as a woman's, but it is there. New thoughts, new priorities, new emotions, new love—all there and hardwired by nature.

This is tremendously important news for two reasons. First, given the way American culture operates, science will slowly start to fill in the story of fatherhood with discoveries, and what will be revealed about families and men's role in reproduction and family life will be scientifically and philosophically profound, as well as poetic. The rudiments of these ideas are already powerful as metaphors. Men experiencing a permanent emotional transformation. The hormonal and symbolic synchronization and communication that takes place between mates. The importance of reinforcing the pair bond during pregnancy. A male partner's effect on the timing, duration, and ease of labor and delivery. The critical importance of paternal investment. These are potentially validating ideas that hint at how connected men are to the undiscovered story of the family. Ironically these million-year-old developments—the idea that motherhood and fatherhood arose as a dialog between the sexes over evolutionary time—may also alter our view of other contemporary roles: for example, complementing, demystifying, and rewriting notions of motherhood.

The other much more immediate and useful development is personal. The idea of transformation—perhaps the most powerful idea humans have—can give men a foothold in a confusing new world. I think it's important to realize that a good part of what gives motherhood its power to women is not the selfless love of another, but that motherhood is an opportunity to know and love a transformed self. When you become a mother you are reborn, and part of life becomes the investigation of that reality. Men also have this opportunity, for there is nothing more inclusive than the idea of transformation. This idea that has been lost symbolically has now been rediscovered biologically, giving men an important new tool and stake in fatherhood and parenthood—the knowledge that they, too, have a new world within to explore.

I'm downstairs making breakfast when I hear giggling coming from the bedroom. I run up the stairs two at a time to investigate and find Julie in bed with Olivia. They are giggling over one of Olivia's books. Olivia is three now and angelic, as three-year-olds are. I beam down on them. Olivia turns to me and opens her mouth. I await some loving pearl.

"Go away, Daddy, I don't want you here."

Bonding may be instinctual, but parenting is not. Every morning I awake to invent myself as a father, and nothing about it has come easily or naturally for me. Every day is a test, a trial, a trove of new mistakes. I often feel I have to earn trust every day. Part of it is not my fault. Being asked to step in and take on a new role demands improvisation. The trouble is, while improvisation can be exciting it is never reliable. Just ask my partner.

This idea of having another opportunity to explore the self is not for the fainthearted. I could fill a book with my shortcomings. Parenting demands consistency, tolerance, patience, and attention to detail—everything that I am bad at. Once, before Olivia arrived, I had imagined that I would be the greatest of fathers. Now that reality has arrived I have to say that I am usually a good father, sometimes merely an okay father, and still not a great one.

Occasionally in moments of reflection I say to myself, "Be careful what you wish for." Parenthood has given me the paradox of myself. I had once imagined that fatherhood would present me with the opportunity to be the protean man, the Ulysses of the home, capable of taking on many different forms and guises, a man the equal of every challenge. What I forgot was Ulysses was probably the most famously absent father of all time, and his wanderings are perhaps nothing more than a parable of a man's unconscious unwillingness to return home.

What disappoints me the most is my own resistance to learning. You would think that someone who reads and writes for a living would absorb and evaluate as many strategies as possible, and yet the biggest fights of our postpartum marriage involve the same theme: Why am I so resistant to learning? Take, for example, parenting books. You would think that I would read forty-odd pages to save my marriage and learn something, but that would mean taking off my cowboy boots for a moment to listen.

What I'm talking about here is not failure, but the unexpected encounter with limitations. The realization that I'm still dealing with the surface of things, the surface of my self. The recognition that one is not as deep as one might think or pretend.

Luckily, Olivia is only three, and there is time to improve.

Then there are the days of pure grace when I put it all together and seem perfect for the job. Like the time during Olivia's early toilet training when she informed us—in the middle of a Laura Ashley sale in the middle of posh Southampton—that she had to poop. You can buy just about any extravagance you want in Southampton, but a place for your child to shit is not one of them. Judging from Olivia's squirm rate I figured we had about forty-five seconds. Julie looked up at me, but I was already gone. In one motion I had scooped up Olivia and whisked her away to the back of the store to the ladies' dressing room along with the white plastic potty insert that I had thought to bring along.

There in a quiet corner I plopped her down and shielded her from view with my body while she squatted. A long minute later it was over. I picked her up and strode as quickly as I could through the store-long gauntlet, smiling all the way, the insert with its brown cargo tucked carefully behind me. The scent of her fresh stool wafting about the absurd clothing and the milling bargain-hunters was headier than violets.

Outside both of us laughed, and Olivia thanked me. It was a real father and daughter moment.

·   ·   ·

While improvisation is unreliable, it is also exhilarating. Like being at the door of an airplane, staring out at the curvature of space and the earth below.

The Huaoroni of the Amazon had it just about right. For them, having a child *creates* the actual marriage. Wife and husband are reborn as mother and father during the birth process. The rituals that both husband and wife go through during the birth process are in essence a second marriage.

I have felt this way since the middle of Julie's pregnancy, when I finally "got" what was going on, and now it is even more true. Being forced to make things up as we go along, to invent, to create, to cobble together has also given us a chance to write the true story of our marriage. This, I now realize, was what Julie and I intended all along when we chose to be parents. To jump through the slick, ambivalent surface of contemporary life into meaningfulness. To live lives of gravity.

Almost every day of Olivia's life, we've had something to put down into the family legend. Nursing Julie through postpartum depression. Taking turns through winter nights with a colicky baby strapped to our chests, plodding the miles to sleep. Holding each other for two hours the first time we tried to "Ferberize"* Olivia. Saving Olivia from choking on her first birthday—a malignant pellet of chicken bone popping into Julie's hand as I whacked Olivia on the back.

This narrative that began in pregnancy is the creation story of our marriage and the center of gravity of our new lives. It's also what we refer to when we can't keep our symbolic lives straight.

---

*Refers to techniques developed by Richard Ferber, M.D., to get a child to sleep on its own.

About one thing we agree without question. Both of us wish for Olivia a selfhood of her own choosing. It is our most cherished idea, the most important idea of our marriage. If there is one thing in the world that gives me hope, it is the knowledge that from the very beginning, from the very moment when she left Julie's womb and entered the world, Olivia has always been her own person.

There is one story about her that sums up much of what I feel about my role in her life. Once when she was about eighteen months old and had just learned to walk we took her with us to dinner at a Japanese restaurant. After dinner we step out onto the street and head home. Olivia takes off. Ever since she learned to walk, she has preferred to run. After a few calls of protest, we are quickly after her.

At the first cross street, there are no cars coming, so I let her cross, running. The blocks pass. Sometimes Julie scoots ahead of her, scouting for cars. Sometimes I signal to make sure they stop. Sometimes I pick Olivia up and whisk her across and set her back down before she can protest. Mostly I follow a few steps behind.

She runs on. Past the Arab livery drivers who look up from their storefront card game and cheer her on. Past the Korean green market where a startled grocer moves his sidewalk cartons aside so she can pass. Past the ice cream store where a group of teenage girls point and twitter in amazement. Past the many faceless passersby who turn and whisper, "Look at that little girl!" The little girl whose face is an expression of boundless, fearless joy.

By later calculation, she runs almost a half-mile before she trips on a crack in the sidewalk and falls onto her hands. She cries, as much out of exhaustion as pain. I comfort her, stroking the back of her head as she buries her face in my shoulder.

Every time I remember this story I see the future. I know there will be times when I should clear the way, and times when I should get the hell out of the way. Knowing which is required will be the art of being Olivia's father. And when I remember this story I also remember a promise I made to myself way back when during Julie's pregnancy.

Those beautiful early days when I made a commitment to follow as well as lead.

INDEX

INDEX